MW01673437

entwined

A STORY OF *WAVERING* FAITH AND BEAUTIFUL MIRACLES

Khalie A. Perez

CLC Publishing

Copyright © 2021 by Khalie Perez

All rights reserved. No part of this book may be used or reproduced in any manner whatsoever without written permission of the author.

Published by CLC Publishing, LLC.
Mustang, OK 73064

Printed in the United States of America

Book Design by Shannon Whittington
Cover Image by Scantling Photography
Back Cover Photo by Kalee Isenhour

ISBN: 978-1-7363318-1-1

Health/Pregnancy and Childbirth

1

Ever since I was a little girl, I wanted children. I can remember being twelve years old and deciding that I'd be having triplets when I was older. Clearly, I didn't completely understand how the whole baby thing worked. I just knew that it would be really awesome to have three babies all at the same time. I even went as far as picking out their names. Get ready for this... April, May and June. How perfect, right?! I'll wait while you try and think of better names. It's hard, right?!

As I got older and slightly wiser, the thought of having triplets started to feel like it would be a little too overwhelming. So instead, I chose the more common scenario. I'd get married, have two kids, a dog, plus a white picket fence. That was the picture-perfect dream that I dreamt for myself. Easy peasy, lemon squeezy. But you know, sometimes life throws buckets and buckets and then some more buckets of lemons at you. So, you grab the sugar, put on your apron, and make the best dang lemonade in all the land.

In my picture-perfect life, I'd have a boy and a girl. I imagined what life would be like and the challenges that having one of each would bring. Even though I wanted both, I wanted my first to be a girl. I wanted to have someone that was a mini version of myself (as scary as that sounds). I wanted to do all the girly things that you do with daughters; paint our nails, play dress up, talk about boys, every last bit of it.

I'm going to tell you a little bit about me because, obviously, I'm writing this book and maybe it'll give you a little glimpse into the life I'm living. First off, my name is Khalie, pronounced *Callie*, or you know, *Cali* like California. It is phonetically correct and there is not a single person that can tell me otherwise. My mom loved names, and names with unique spellings. That's where I got my obsession.

I love cooking for people. It's like my love language. I even go as far as making their plates. I'm not sure when or why I ever started that. My husband used to tell me all the time, "Khalie, I can make my own plate you know." But through the years, he's given up and sits at the table waiting for his plate and says thank you when I put it in front of him. I promise I am not one of those old-fashioned wives from decades ago that have dinner on the table as soon as he walks through the door. It's just as simple as me showing love through food.

A hobby that I've really started loving in the past year or so is quilting. It's proven to be a challenge but having it finished is such a feeling of accomplishment, especially since I've been known to lose interest rather quickly. I'm currently on a mission to make all of my favorite people their own handmade quilt. It's a bit ambitious, but what's life without goals?

2

Parents. We all have them, right? Whether they're good, bad or indifferent, we have them. Me though, I have the absolute best parents in the world. Four total parents to be exact. I'm about 99.9% positive that God gave me four parents because He knew it would be a combined effort made by all of them to raise me. I still think that after 35 years, they're still raising me. When I say that I was a handful, that's not a dramatic statement but more of an understatement. I was difficult in every possible sense of the word. I had to ALWAYS get my way and I mean always. Once, when I was around 3 years old, I saw a phone in a store and just had to have it. My dad leaned down to tell me that I wasn't going to get the phone and I bit his ear. There was blood. I mean it when I say I had more sass and attitude than four high school girls combined all by the time I was two. I probably have just a bit of that sass left, but I like to think that I've mellowed out some; although my family may (and probably does) think otherwise.

Throughout my teenage years, I was still quite a mess. I know that most teenagers cause at least some kind of trouble, but I was on a whole other level, like master level. I never snuck out or did any of the "typical" teenage rebellious things though. I was way more of the have-the-worst-possible-attitude, didn't know how to speak my mind in a nice way, kind of teenager. Other than talking a lot in class, I was a good student. Unfortunately, that meant most of my attitude was directed toward my family. They loved me through it though, and to this day I only remember being super grounded once. That ordeal lasted an entire month. A month is like an eternity for a teenager. Oh, and then there was the one time that they took me to get a "new to me" car, and I got to test drive it home. It was a green Honda Civic and I wanted it like I never wanted anything before. I was so excited to be turning 16 and to be getting a new car. But in typical Khalie fashion, I had an attitude about who knows what. I'm pretty sure that it was over something dumb and my dumb attitude prompted a quick trip back to the dealership the next day where I left that beautiful green, great gas milage car right there on the lot.

Little back story: My mom and dad divorced when I was two. I don't remember too much about life when it was just the three of us though. About the only thing I remember is that they would hold my hands in a parking lot and swing me by my arms, which I thought was absolutely the most fun thing ever. I'd like to mention that I was also born on my mom and dad's anniversary; how many people can say that? Thankfully, they still liked each other because they'd never be able to forget what day they were married unless they forgot my birthday and that would just be wrong.

My dad married my bonus mom when I was around three and my mom married my bonus dad when I was twelve. All four of my parents have gotten along ever since I can remember. I'm sure there was a learning curve of some sort in the early stages, but I didn't really notice. My mom and bonus mom even got each other Christmas presents, would talk often, and just last year the three of us took a quilting class together (we would even ride together and have brunch before). Oh, I can't forget that I got to have both of them with me when I picked out my wedding dress. Apparently, that doesn't happen too often because I remember the sales lady asking her co-workers if they could believe that those two were my mom and stepmom.

My dad and bonus dad get along, too. So much so that when I got married my dad made sure that I was having my bonus dad walk me down the aisle with him. I'm telling you that they get along so well that they could all sit down together and write their own book about co-parenting and it would be a bestseller; I'm sure of it.

Birthdays, holidays, and any and all other events were smooth sailing. There was never any drama like you hear about with other families. I was able to enjoy all my family together on many different occasions and it was like we were all one big happy family. I think that it's so important for a child to see their parents get along despite divorce. Having a healthy relationship between everyone involved can really shape the child when it comes to their own future relationships. I'll spare you from having to read my soapbox but know this: I am the only child from my mom and dad's marriage. That marriage ended over 30 years ago. There was no reason that they HAD to continue talking after I turned 18, but they did. All my parents were and continued to be friends even as I became an adult.

My bonus mom shared this story with me a few months ago... She said that at my high school graduation party, her and my mom were standing outside, and my bonus mom said, "It's not over, is it?" and my mom looked at her and said, "No, she's ours."

As a child, I felt loved by all of them equally. As an adult, going through the ups and downs of life, I was able to have the four of them by my side no matter what was going on. They are a united front. When there was any kind of bad news, they would all be there to tell me together. I wish that I could fully paint a picture of how incredibly blessed I am to have them as parents. There was never a question that my parents loved and respected each other, too. They were teammates when it came to raising me and having me as their daughter.

My mom had a heart of gold. She lived her life serving others. Whether it was when she was teaching her elementary students, giving to those in need, or taking care of her family, she did it with a selfless heart. My mom was strict but only when she needed to be. She taught me to speak my mind (I may have taken that a little too literally). My mom taught me how to be a mom. I will never come close to her as a mother, but I strive to be just as close as I can. She was loving, she was strong, she was creative, she was patient and every other good thing you can think of.

One thing that my mom and I shared was our love to serve others. She taught me how to give and I live my life trying to be just as giving as she was. She was and will always be the best mom and Lolli that the world's ever seen. My mom was one of a kind. God gave us a mom and Lolli worth more than jewels when he gave us her.

My dad. Whew, now he is a character. He is the absolute best at making up stories that involve all sorts of crazy scenarios. It wouldn't be too much for him to say that he wrangled up a one-eyed crocodile, wrestled it to the ground and served it for supper and did it all with his hands behind his back. He likes to pick on you, but that's how you know he loves you. My dad is stubborn, Mr. Fix It, hard-headed, the hardest worker, hilarious, and loves his family like nothing else. I think I get my sense of humor and weirdness from him. He is the world's best dad and granddad and we are so thankful he's ours.

My bonus mom means so much to me. Stepping in to help raise a child can be overwhelming. She has always made me feel like I was her daughter, and I have never doubted her love for me. She would make my clothes, she would braid my hair (thanks to her and her French braids, I'm not tender headed), teach me how to cook, and she's currently teaching me how to quilt. She is loving, caring, patient, and so many more wonderful things. When I don't know what to do or am worried, she has a calming perspective to give. She is the greatest. I couldn't have asked for a better bonus mom and Gramms than her.

My bonus dad is likely the most understanding and rational person on the planet. Even when it came to me and my antics, he was calm and never judged me. I can maybe count on three fingers how many times I have seen him truly angry, and that's stretching it. He always has advice worth hearing and helps you to see things differently, usually in a better way. He is logical, knows a little about a lot of things, patient, works hard and does everything for his family. There's not a greater bonus dad or Pops on the planet.

I've been blessed with five siblings that are all younger than me. I have three brothers and two sisters. Two of my brothers are four years younger than me. I have a brother and a sister that are 13 years younger than me and my other sister is 12 years younger. None are twins though, and I'll let you try and figure that out. I wish I could say because I'm the oldest I'm the wisest, but that's far from the truth. They each bring something of their own into my life: Some crazy, some yelling, some competitiveness but more than anything, love. I hope when they look at my life, they can take the good parts and apply them to their own lives while also learning from the many, and I mean *many*, mistakes I've made. I would like to think that I made all my mistakes on their behalf so they wouldn't have to. I think it goes with the whole protective older sister thing, saving them from themselves and all.

3

I started dating my first husband when I was twenty. We eventually got married when I was twenty-three. The point of me telling you all that is mostly irrelevant (but kind of not) because it was during this time in my life that I was told that it may be difficult for me to have children. I don't think that I was ever formally diagnosed, but I was told by a doctor that I had polycystic ovary syndrome (PCOS).

We had been trying for over a year and a half, I believe, before we decided that I would begin taking medication to increase my chances of becoming pregnant. I kid you not that it wasn't even two months after I started taking it that he told me he wanted a divorce. There was no super dramatic scandal or some secret life either of us were living. Nothing that would lead to a Lifetime movie either. We just weren't right for each other and as cliché as that sounds, it's the truth. We had a drama free split and then that chapter was closed.

I struggled with the divorce. It wasn't because I felt like we were supposed to be together but more so that I thought that I was getting closer to my dream of having a family and then it vanished, and I didn't even see it coming. Those five or so years we were together were years that I would never get back and that made me angry and sad at the same time. I wanted nothing more than to have a family, and at that point in my life, it felt like it was further away than ever. I had to start all the way over. I had to make the effort to date again plus I had to find someone that would put up with me enough to marry me, and that in itself was a big ask.

I was really at a crossroads during this whole time. While I was married, I was also going to school for a social work degree. At the time of my divorce, I was doing my practicum at the same place that my ex-husband worked, Children's Hospital. Remember when I said that I had a bit of an attitude? Well, I think that my ex-husband wanted to prevent me from making a scene, so he asked (more so informed me that I had to) find another place to do my practicum. So, I was going through a divorce while trying to maintain my college requirements. It was a lot. It felt like I was just barely hanging on. Thankfully though, I had a lot of support to get me through to the other side of the whole thing.

I finally started using the time after my divorce to figure out what I wanted out of my new life. I spent time with my friends, met new friends, went to a whole lot of concerts and found out that I could and would be okay on my own. I didn't have to have all the answers as to what my life would look like. Before all of this happened, I had always thought that I would get married at 22, have children by the time that I was 24 and I would be set. Here I was though: single, 25 and completely starting over but that was okay; I'd be okay.

4

A year or two after my divorce, I met David at a Red Dirt concert. This concert lasted three nights. No, it wasn't like a rage or whatever those things are called that never end. I actually did go home and sleep.

David and I met on the first night. The main concert was over, and another band was playing inside. I walked up to him as confidently as I could and of all things, I told him that I didn't like his hat. In my defense it was a Boston Red Sox hat and I'm a Texas Rangers fan through and through. I'd spent my childhood going to Ranger games.

David and I talked for a few minutes before he went on his way and I thought to myself, "Ok, see ya later." Let me remind you that my name is quite uniquely spelled. That night or maybe the next day, I got a friend request from David. He'd remembered how to spell my name! I later learned he's the king of remembering random things.

I skipped the second night of the concert but made it back the third night. I actually hadn't planned on going that third night, but my friend gave me her VIP tickets and I wasn't about to turn down a good time. So, there I was enjoying the music and who do I see in the endless mass of people? You guessed it. David. There he was, walking right past me. I grabbed him by the arm and told him that he should hang out with us (because clearly, I was more fun than whatever he had going on).

We spent the rest of the night enjoying the music, talking and having a good time. The next day he treated me to lunch. I remember that afternoon when I got home, I already knew that I wanted to see him again. So, I broke all the dating rules and invited him to hang out that evening.

In full disclosure, I asked him if he wanted to come to a party. Little did he know that when he got there, I was the party. He still says I tricked him and that he probably wouldn't have come if he had known it was just going to be me. A tad bit rude because I'm super fun. Anyway, I guess I won him over because we were officially dating a couple of weeks later.

I always wondered when I started dating someone, how the conversation would go once I told them that it may be difficult for me to get pregnant. So even though we hadn't been dating for that long, I decided to get it out of the way. I told David that I had tried having children during my first marriage and wasn't ever able to get pregnant. We didn't talk about it too much and I knew we would just cross that bridge when and if we got there.

We dated for just about two years before he decided that he just couldn't live his life without me, (or maybe I told him to get me the ring I picked out, but either way), we got engaged in December 2014.

Can I just take this time to say that I hadn't had the flu since the fourth grade? I remember it was the fourth grade because while I was out sick with the flu, my class was learning long division. I was never able to catch up and math is still my enemy.

Anyway, that January after we got engaged, I felt like I had that same flu. I was the sickest I had been in decades. I felt horrible for weeks and was starting to get frustrated that I wasn't getting any better. I'm awful when I get sick, almost as bad as a man, but not quite.

When it was clear that I wasn't getting any better, my mom and bonus mom, in separate conversations (but within about a day of each other), suggested that I take a pregnancy test. Quick Fun Fact: those two were known to get me the same presents on occasion. Once they even wore the same Easter Dress. All on accident of course; at least that's what they said. They got along so well that I wouldn't have been surprised if they had planned it.

I wanted to prove that their suggestion that I could be pregnant was wrong, so I took a test. I didn't believe what it said so I took two or three more. Sure enough, they all said the same thing: Pregnant. Positive. Hey, Khalie there's a baby in there. I was shocked. I couldn't believe it. Something that I thought may never happen, was going to happen. David and I were going to be parents. Our lives were about to flip upside down.

5

My first appointment was a family affair. My dad, bonus mom, mom, bonus dad, David and my pregnant self all went to the appointment. I was so nervous leading up to my appointment because I felt like maybe I took the tests wrong somehow. It's not rocket science or anything, but I was certain that it couldn't have been that easy. There was no way that I got pregnant without medical intervention.

When I saw the screen, there was no more doubt. It was real and we had the "Hi, Mom and Dad" ultrasound to prove it. We absolutely couldn't wait to tell all of our family and friends. We bought a picture frame that said *'Our Little Miracle'* on it and placed our proof inside it. We took a picture of the picture and posted it online so that it was official.

I spent the next several weeks almost in denial. It's like I was in a dream and was going to wake up any second. I never in a million years thought that I would be able to get pregnant that easily. As a matter of fact, I told David that I wanted to start "trying to have a baby" so that by the time we got married, I could go to the doctor and say, "I've been trying to get pregnant for a long time and it hasn't worked so how can we make this happen?" I didn't want to waste any time having a family. So, knowing that it took just a few months was surreal.

I know there was a baby in my tummy, and I had zero previous experience of being pregnant, but I felt like I was sicker than any other pregnant woman in the history of the entire universe had ever been.

A few weeks later we went to the appointment where they determine your due date. My mom and David were there with me. She started the ultrasound and a few seconds later asked how I had been feeling. I kind of laughed, but was totally serious, when I told her that I always felt sick, sicker than what I felt was normal. Like I had a reference, right? She laughed and said that she was sure I was feeling sick because there were actually two babies on the way.

Two babies. Two babies, not one. Excuse me? What did you just say? I had hit a new stage of denial. I couldn't believe it. I will go on, not too much of a limb, and say that David and my mom were just as shocked as I was.

I immediately called my bonus mom while I was still laying on the table because she needed to hear the news ASAP. I remember the laughing and overall joy from her and my mom both. My bonus mom told me later that when I had called her with the news, she was running happily around her office like a teenager at a Beatles Concert. Twins wasn't too far off from triplets, but I was still short a June so my brilliant trio of names would have to wait (and the world rejoiced).

Soon after the shock (kind of, but not really) wore off, we began thinking about how expensive it was going to be to have two babies at one time. Costs of diapers, car seats, cribs, daycare and all things baby. Future vehicle costs, having two kids in college at the same time, the whole shebang. Having a baby isn't cheap and now we were having two. How in the world were we going to have two babies at the same time? How were we going to pay for two babies at the same time? I didn't have a job during this time and even if I did go back to work, it would be as a social worker and it's not like they're paid enough.

We had all of the logical thoughts, but we also had fears. The normal twin pregnancy ones like twin-to-twin transfusion, miscarriage, prematurity, etc. We didn't dwell too much on the fears, though, because we were so excited to be parents and we couldn't wait to meet our babies.

My original OB referred us to a doctor that specialized in twin pregnancies at a Perinatal Office. We weren't referred to him because she saw anything wrong in the ultrasounds, but because his specialty was twin pregnancies.

Our first appointment with that doctor was set for four weeks later at which we would be having our gender ultrasound. I spent those next few weeks basking in the thought of how life changing this all was. Dreaming about what their nursery would look like and of course coming up with a stellar list of names because names are like a hobby for me. I was so excited that I couldn't think about anything else. I loved spending time planning their arrival. I loved every second of those dreams.

6

Gender reveals are quite a thing and we wanted to be cool and have one too. We couldn't wait to find out, with our family and friends, what our sweet babes were. My mom, bonus mom and I started planning the party pretty quickly. We went out to dinner one night and started planning. We talked about what food and drinks we would have and all the other details that would make this the perfect party to find out if we were having boys, girls or one of each. We even went as far as writing a cute little poem that we used on the homemade invitations. Once the guest list was complete, the invitations were sent on their way. The party was going to be amazing.

It seemed like it took forever to get to 18 weeks, but I finally made it. We woke up so excited to find out what we would be having. My mom, bonus mom, and David's mom were there with us at the appointment. Once we got to the doctor's office, we anxiously waited for them to call my name and take us back to our room.

The ultrasound technician came in and began the ultrasound. I remember our moms looking at the screen as the tech was rolling that machine over my belly. David and I had already decided that we were going to wait to find out what we were having until the gender reveal party, so we weren't looking.

The room was so quiet, eerily quiet. I had the strangest feeling and it scared me because I should have been excited to finally learn what they were. I remember looking at my mom and asking her why it was so quiet. She reassured me that the tech was just doing her job and that I shouldn't worry.

I can't explain why but I started crying, tears flowing uncontrollably, and at that point, I didn't have a reason other than maybe my motherly intuition was kicking in. After a few minutes the tech stood up, said she was having a hard time finding the genders, and was going to go get the doctor.

I was confused. Why wasn't she able to see the genders? What was going on with my babies? Were they even alive? I had no idea what was going on. I just laid there trying to tell myself that everything was ok, even though that's not even close to how I felt.

Finally, the tech and doctor were in the room. The doctor didn't hesitate to tell us what he saw on the ultrasound. He told us that there was a complication and that the twins were conjoined. Conjoined? Why? How? I didn't know how to process what he was saying. He told us that he had only seen this one other time in his twenty-year career and that those twins didn't survive past 25 weeks in utero.

I knew what he meant by that statement. Conjoined twins are rare, and he was letting me (us) know that it's likely that they wouldn't survive. I know that he was doing his job as a doctor, but the way he said it was so cold. I felt like he was already giving our twins a death sentence. I'm sure that I would've been worried and scared no matter how he gave us the information, but I think that he could have done it with a little compassion.

For a doctor, giving news to families can be routine. For us, the news he gave us would change our lives forever. It would have been nice if he would have given us a little bit of hope. Even if he had just reminded us in that very moment there were still two very strong hearts beating.

Everything after the conjoined twin part was such a blur and I don't remember most of it. He was saying words, but I couldn't hear him or maybe I didn't want to hear him. Maybe I was trying to tell myself that this wasn't happening. Our babies were going to be fine and live a happy and healthy life.

The few parts that I do remember him saying were that Baby A had a clubbed foot and that they may be sharing their liver or kidney. Because of how they were positioned, they couldn't tell us the gender, but being conjoined twins did mean that they were identical. Oh, and somewhere in there I remember that he mentioned termination. He really did just lay it all out there.

I remember David sitting on the floor sobbing with his head down and hands covering his face. I had never seen him like that. It was hard to see the man I loved so scared of losing our babies. There wasn't anything that we could say to each other that would make it all ok. There wasn't a way to make this all go away. It was as if the world had just ended at that moment and to us, it had.

The doctor told us that we could wait in the room until I felt like I could walk out. I didn't want to move. My world stopped in that room and I didn't want to face life if I didn't have my babies with me. I felt like I wasn't going to make it another second much less the rest of my pregnancy.

We left that office in pieces. All the dreams we had for our little family, shattered in the span of a few seconds. The pain that I felt is something that I will never be able to adequately describe. There are no words in any dictionary that could describe how crushed my soul was from that day on and the months that followed. There's no way that I could've prepared myself to hear that I might not be bringing our babies home. Even thinking about the complications regarding twin pregnancies, not in a million or even a billion years would I have ever thought that they would be conjoined. But they were, and I couldn't do anything to fix it.

The car ride home was hard. Our family and friends were waiting to hear about how the appointment went. Now, we were heading home to share devastating news with them. How was I going to be able to even speak the words the doctor shared with us?

I remember riding home from the appointment laying my head down, still sobbing, and asking my family what I had done wrong. Why were our babies this way? What did I ever do that would make God do this to our family? Why after all these years of looking forward to having children would this be the way that I would become a mother? How could I save them?

We had to cancel the gender reveal party, for obvious reasons. You can't really have a gender reveal party when you don't know what genders to reveal. Cancelling the party made it feel even more real for me. The party was going to be our first celebration with our family and friends, and we weren't able to have it. I'm sure that when my mom and bonus mom let everyone know that there was no longer going to be a party, there was some kind of explanation that happened. Slowly but surely, people were going to start learning about what was going on with our babies.

We were overwhelmed by sympathy and kind words. For me, the fact that I needed that type of support was a constant reminder of the gravity of our situation. Even the kindest words and prayers offered were still difficult to hear. Each conversation brought me back to the moment when my world turned upside down. With every new person that I would talk to, it was as if I were reliving the day that we had found out that the twins were conjoined. They would ask questions and I couldn't give them any answers. I couldn't tell them what they shared or if they were going to live.

There were some that were hopeful and would tell me they believed everything would be okay, but it sure didn't feel like it.

7

I'm not sure any expectant mother can prepare herself to hear that abortion is an option. How does one handle hearing those words come out of the mouth of a medical professional? One that has spent years in medical school and even longer practicing medicine.

I am about to be really real here, so be kind. I have my beliefs on abortion, just like anyone else. For me, abortion would never be a choice that I would personally make for myself. However, I would be lying if I said that there wasn't a split second when the doctor told us the news, that I didn't think in my head that it may be the easier way to go.

I didn't know what the next few months would bring. I was scared that I wouldn't be able to make it if I lost them naturally, so maybe I should just get it over with. What kind of mom was I to even think that? How could I give up on my children?

Even though I had those thoughts for only a few seconds, it's still hard to think about. I feel guilty that those thoughts even crossed my mind. I felt so powerless and helpless, and maybe I thought that I would be making it easier on all of us if I decided to end my pregnancy. Whatever the reason, to this day I still haven't forgiven myself for even considering it for those few seconds.

It's as if all of the joy I felt from those first weeks, finding out that I was pregnant and then finding out that I was pregnant with twins, never even existed. I could no longer dream about their nursery or add names to my list. I went from wondering their genders, to wondering if they were going to survive.

From that point on, I couldn't think about the future. The only thing that I could think about was how I was going to make it through each day. I would wake up weeping, nearly having a panic attack most nights. I was so afraid to go to sleep because I knew that when I woke up, it was going to be another long day of feeling like I was barely surviving.

What I am about to reveal to you is important. As a matter of fact, it's most likely the most personal information that I could possibly share. The reason that I want to share this with you is because I feel like these feelings/behaviors/tendencies that I have play a huge role in my story.

I have suffered from depression, obsessive compulsive disorder, anxiety, and severe highs/lows, since my teenage years and probably even earlier.

When I say I suffer from depression, I'm not talking about what I like to call, situational depression. I am talking about depression that comes out of nowhere and that doesn't really have a rhyme or reason. Apparently, I don't do things halfway because I also have "situational depression" which I describe as depression being triggered by an event or incident in life.

When I say I have OCD, I don't mean in the way that people casually and jokingly say they have OCD, like having to have their towels folded a certain way. I'm talking the whole nine yards. The hand washing, the lock checking and so many other quirks that it would take a whole other book to write about.

The anxiety that I have in my daily life causes the OCD tendencies and the whole thing is a vicious cycle. The highs and lows are just another piece in my mental health puzzle. They aren't fun and often come at the expense of my family.

What I want to make crystal clear is that there is no shame in seeking professional help. Finding people that are trained to guide you through those obstacles and hurdles so you don't have to navigate them alone is the best thing you can do for yourself. I don't want to jump on a soapbox, because that would make this book even longer, but I do want to let those that need to hear it know that you're not alone. Seek help, you deserve it.

Because of my mental health, the days that followed were more of the same. A complete and total blur. I was basically waking up each day wanting the day to be over. I wasn't really living, I was existing. I didn't want to do anything. I couldn't do anything. My thoughts were constantly about what was going to happen to our babies. I would spend so many hours searching online for statistics of conjoined twins. I was desperately trying to find conjoined twins that made it to delivery and separation. My thoughts and searches almost debilitated me. I was so wrapped up in all of the negative outcomes, that I could barely function.

We were staying at my mom's house during this time because before I got pregnant, we were living in an apartment on the third floor. Can you believe that I requested the third floor? All because I didn't want to hear people stomping around above me. I hadn't really factored in carrying groceries up three flights of stairs or being pregnant. I wish that I could tell you that I thought it was good exercise but, no, it was plain awful.

While we were staying with my parents, we were in the process of remodeling our condo that we would eventually be moving into. It was good that we were staying with my parents because after a few days, David had to go back to work and there was no way that I could handle being by myself for any amount of time.

I could hardly take a shower. I remember that after my showers, my mom would brush, dry and straighten my hair. I just didn't have the energy to do it. I didn't even want to eat. The simplest, daily things turned out to be things that were barely attainable for me. The depression was so deep that I thought I would live in that darkness for the rest of my life. I thought I knew the extent of what depression looked like but really, I had no clue. This was unlike any other depression I had ever felt before and it was scary. I was scared that the depression would never leave, and I would never be able to find joy again.

8

We had appointments every single week. On days that we would go to those appointments, I was physically ill before we left because I didn't know if when we got there, I would get to hear their heartbeats. I didn't know if when I looked up, I would get to see my babies moving on the screen. I was terrified that when they started the ultrasound that they would have to tell me that they didn't make it. The appointments rarely gave us new information. Sometimes they were able to tell us what the twins didn't share, but they weren't ever positive about what it was they were actually sharing.

The doctor told us that at 25 weeks we would be transferred to Children's Hospital because at that time, the babies would be viable. There we would be seen at the Prenatal Diagnostic Center at Children's because they were equipped to handle my high-risk pregnancy.

We left each appointment holding on to the heartbeats that we heard to get us through until the next appointment. The ultrasound pictures we would get were so hard for me to look at. Not because they were conjoined, but because I didn't know if the babies I was looking at would even make it through the day, much less the rest of the pregnancy. I would look at them for a few minutes and then put them away where I wouldn't see them again.

Remember how I told you that names were my thing? I was now trying to name my children who I didn't know would ever be able to hear me say those names. Not only that, but we had to pick out four first names and four middle names. The other issue was that David and I couldn't agree on too many names. We finally decided that he would choose a first name and I would choose a first and both middle names because clearly it's only fair since they would have his last name. That was and continues to be my logic to this day. He says that they'll only have his last name until, if and when they get married so if we have another child, I told him he can choose. Thankfully, he has good taste so I'm not too worried.

I could hardly go anywhere because the thought of seeing a pregnant woman was enough to trigger a panic attack. As hard as it is to be this honest and share this with you, I was jealous.

Jealous of other people's happiness. Jealous of life still going on for everyone else while I was just barely hanging on. I was emotionally and mentally drained. Each day was like I was waking up for battle: Battling statistics, depression, anxiety and the most intense fear that I've ever known. During those days my prayer was this: God, if these babies aren't going to make it, please take them now. I don't want to go on with this just to lose them in the end. It breaks my heart to write those words, but it's my truth. I felt that God would be doing me a favor if He would just take them while I was pregnant so that they wouldn't suffer once they came into the world.

You see people go through unimaginable circumstances, complete heartache and you see them do it with grace. They are praying and thanking God for His blessings and all that He's done for them. I've seen pregnant women go on trips knowing that it would be the only trip that they would go on with their child. I wish I could say that I kept my faith intact during this time but that would not even be anywhere near the truth. I am so grateful for my sweet photographer friend who reached out to me and asked if she could take my maternity pictures. I couldn't bring myself to plan the pictures, it's as if I wanted no reminder of my pregnancy. Thankfully, she captured those babies in my tummy and I will cherish those pictures for the rest of my life.

I didn't buy anything for the twins while I was pregnant. I didn't buy cute little outfits, the perfect swaddling blankets or the cuddliest teddy bears. I didn't pick out cribs or car seats. Some moms that are told that their child/children will most likely not survive, buy an outfit for their delivery or have special items made for their birth so they could have those as a reminder of their sweet babies. I was not one of those moms. I couldn't begin to make myself buy or make things for them, when I was almost positive that they weren't going to survive.

I went to see my original OB after a few weeks of seeing the Perinatal Doctor. When I went to see her, she told me that she wanted me to go ahead and see the doctors at Children's Hospital because in her opinion, babies are viable at 24 weeks.

Previously, I had set week 25 as a big milestone for the babies because I remembered that doctor telling me that the other set of conjoined twins that he had seen didn't make it past 25 weeks. When my original OB said that she wanted us to go to Children's at 24 weeks, I made that another milestone. I still kept the 25 weeks milestone because if they made it to that week, they would be showing that doctor not to count them out.

The days somehow kept coming and somehow, I was making it through them as I waited for week 24. Nothing much changed as I was waiting to get to Children's other than those babies kept growing and letting us hear those beautiful heartbeats.

9

Once we finally made it to Children's, it instantly felt different than all the other appointments we had in the past. There was a tech who did the initial ultrasound and I just laid there silently. I remember that I really liked her, and that she did her best to help keep my spirits up as much as she could. I don't know if dread is the right word to describe my feelings toward these appointments, because it seems wrong to say, but they were never appointments filled with any excitement. The only joyous feeling I had was knowing that there were still heartbeats. Even hearing those heartbeats, was incredibly difficult because I didn't know how long I would get to hear them.

I met my new OB during this appointment too. Initially, I was concerned about how young I believed her to be. Would she really be able to handle this? I just added that to my ever-growing list of fears. A pediatric surgeon also joined us during that appointment. He sat down and started looking at the ultrasound on the screen. I continued to lay there quietly. I would hear him say to the doctor and tech, “This is good.” I would hear comments like that every few seconds. Finally, I looked over to him and said, “What about this is good?” I couldn’t imagine that after all of my research and seeing statistics that there was anything positive about our situation. He told us that they were joined at the abdomen and that he would be able to separate them. I even think at some point I heard him say, “I can do this.” That right there was the first positive thing said to us by any medical professional since we began our journey. He wasn’t able to tell us exactly what they shared or their gender, but he did give us a small sense of hope. That itty bitty amount of hope that he gave me, helped me through my darkest days.

Days went by just as they had been, mostly. I didn’t talk to my friends often. I couldn’t. This was hard for me because I’ve been blessed with the same circle of friends since elementary school. Friends that I talked to often even after over 25 years of friendship. I didn’t know how to talk about anything other than what I was going through, and I didn’t feel like it was fair for them to have to hear my pain. To see me in the state that I was in and didn't know if I would ever get out of, was not something that I wanted them to see. Even though I didn't talk to them much during my pregnancy, I will always remember the hope that they had for the babies. Their encouraging words and how they reminded me that God is always in control. My friends are one in a million and I'm blessed to have them.

So many women have cravings and get to use the guilt free card about eating anything and everything they want, and why wouldn't they? Growing a human is hard work. Eating for me was so incredibly hard. I tried to eat fruits and vegetables, which was hard because my idea of healthy eating is fruit-flavored sweets and the only vegetables I care about are potatoes. Baked potatoes to be exact, with tons of cheese, bacon and more sour cream than should ever be allowed. Potatoes are still a staple food group for me these days. I wanted to do what was best for the babies but struggling with depression and anxiety made it tough. I only gained 30lbs during my pregnancy, but I did my best to be as healthy as I could be for the two of them.

The following weeks were filled with more ultrasounds and testing. One of those tests was the echo fetal cardiology appointment. This was an appointment where they would look at the twins' hearts. Even though I was told during my other appointments that they didn't share a heart, I was still scared that somehow, they got it wrong. Somehow, they missed something. Sharing hearts, as you can conclude, means zero survival rate. The appointment went as well as it could have, and I remember that the doctor took the time to draw out a diagram to help me understand what it was that he saw.

The most important takeaway was that he was certain that they each had their very own heart. As happy as I was to hear that, it was hard to fully rejoice with any good news because the outcome was still unknown and from what I had read, the odds weren't in our favor.

10

One day my parents, David and I went to a local tree farm to pick out trees to plant in the twins' honor. It would be something that we could watch grow over the years and no matter the outcome, we would have them to symbolize our journey. It was that very day that we planted those trees that I finally felt them kick. I was cautiously excited and told my family the news. It was a strange emotion though. On one hand, I was happy that I would be reminded of their presence and that they were alive but at the same time I was scared of what would happen if the kicks stopped coming. I had known in my heart and mind that they had been alive for months but now I was able to feel it. It became even more real for me that day.

I have always been one to seek validation. Not for myself in any kind of way necessarily, more so validation in that things are going to be ok. I know it isn't rational but it's something that gives me peace. I would ask my doctors and the rest of the medical team so many questions. Mostly questions that they couldn't really answer. I would ask them if they thought that the twins would survive? What their life would look like if they did? So many questions and usually the same questions over and over again. There was one doctor, Dr. Williams, that really said something to me that I still think about to this day. He said that in unknown situations only allow yourself to ask four "what-if" questions and after you ask them, that's it. No more what-ifs. That advice can be hard to follow, but it's still something that I remind myself about all these years later.

Let's talk about names again, shall we? I am one of THOSE PEOPLE that won't name my children a name of someone I know. It can't be the same name as someone I went to school with. It can't be a far distant cousin and it most certainly can't be the name of someone famous. There are also things to think about like initials and what the initials spelled out. For instance, our last name is Perez so clearly neither name could start with a P. It drove David bananas but hey, this is something permanent so the decision couldn't and shouldn't be made lightly. Oh, and I'm one who has to know the meanings of names. Even though I know that there are a thousand variations of meanings of each name, I still had to like it. I couldn't have the meaning of their name be something weird, like a wild boar in a meadow or sad prairie flower. I spent hours upon hours, days upon days, weeks upon weeks searching for the perfect names. Everyone had to like them too. I wasn't one of those smart people that kept the names a secret until after the birth and at which point if you criticized the name you were just rude and probably wouldn't be invited to their first birthday party or any after that for that matter. After what seemed like an eternity, we finally picked out names that we loved. If they were boys their names would be Lincoln Andrew and Dawson Leon. David picked out Lincoln and I chose Dawson. The middle names are family names.

If they were girls, one of them would be named Hartlyn Amira. David chose Everlee (I told you he was good) and Ilya would be the middle name. It felt good to finally choose names that we all loved. I will also note that I spend a lot of time picking out pet names and they also have to have middle names. So, believe me when I say that picking out the twins' names was a huge task and one that I was very happy we had accomplished.

11

As the twins grew it became clear that if they did survive birth that they would need special accommodations. The first thing that they would need would be a bed that would hold both of them. In the position that they were in, one would have to be built. It's hard to imagine, and we were constantly trying to draw pictures to get a visual of how they were positioned so that we could understand. The best way that I can describe their position is that they were in almost an X shape facing each other. The next concern was how to keep the baby that was on the top from suffocating the baby on the bottom with their weight. I'm almost positive that it was not in their job description but the maintenance men at the hospital worked hard on making sure that, if need be, our babies would have exactly what they needed after birth. Another concern was how to get the babies oxygen if they needed or anesthesia if they survived long enough to attempt a separation surgery. It was so overwhelming to think about all the things that needed to be in place by the time of delivery. Thankfully, there was a whole team of medical professionals that had a plan and spent long hours practicing how the unique delivery would go.

We continued to make it through each day and each day the fear grew, which seems impossible that I could have been anymore scared, but I was as time went on. Each day that we made it through was another day closer to their delivery. Soon, we would meet with the surgeon that we had met at our first appointment when we got to Children's. During our appointment he talked to us about waiting until they were maybe a month old before planning on separating them. He wanted them to grow as much as they could, giving them the best chance for a successful outcome. Things were getting more and more real.

There came a day where I was in a good amount of pain. I ended up going to the hospital where they told me that I had starting dilating. I stayed in the hospital a couple of nights so that they could monitor any progress. They gave me medicine to try and slow things down because the twins needed to stay in there as we still had several weeks to go, and we were hoping to make it to the scheduled c-section date that was set for 36 weeks.

Thankfully, my body did what we had hoped, and the medication kept them put.

12

I want to share all the feelings that I felt. I want to speak to that mom that is where I was. I want to speak to that mom that has been given that news that their precious child may not make it long in this world. I want to speak to the NICU moms. I want to speak to the moms that have medically complex children. I want them to know that their feelings are valid. So here I go, sharing my most raw and intense feelings in the hopes that it finds the person that needs to hear that they are not alone.

Grief: I was grieving something that hadn't even happened yet. I was already mourning the loss of my children. I was grieving the loss of the life that I had dreamed of and was so excited for. I was grieving all the things that I wouldn't get to experience while I was pregnant: the joy, nesting, baby showers, etc. I was grieving the person that I was before I was pregnant because there was no way that I would ever be that person again. I was grieving in every sense of the word. I hadn't ever grieved something so deeply before.

Anger: During most, (by most I mean all after we found out the news), of my pregnancy, I was angry. I was angry at my body for failing my children. I was angry that God would DO THIS to our family. I was angry that I had waited for years to have a child, only to be faced with the possibility of them not even surviving to birth. I was angry that they may not survive after birth. I was angry that if they did survive birth, that they may not survive the separation surgery. I was angry that if they did survive the separation surgery, that their lives would be filled with pain and hardship. I was angry at just about everything. I wanted so badly to have trust in God's plan, but I didn't like the plan that I believed He had for our family, which was a plan that would leave my heart broken beyond repair. A plan that would turn me into the most bitter person to ever walk the Earth.

Pain: It's hard to even put into words the pain that I felt. I don't think that it's something that I can describe. It's a pain that you won't truly understand unless you've been there. It's like the most horrible pain that you can imagine, plus so much more. I was in pain every single day. Not just physical pain, but emotional pain. Pain that was hard to really grasp and make sense of. Pain that felt like it was suffocating me. A pain that there was no relief for.

I felt out of control. I usually need, or at least feel like I need to be in control of everything in my life, and this was something way beyond my control. I couldn't take a magical pill and make everything ok. I couldn't just go to the doctor and have them "fix it". That was the absolute hardest thing for me, not being able to help my children. Not being able to make everything ok.

Guilt: One of the worst feelings that you can feel. I spent so much of my time questioning what I did wrong. Blaming myself for what my babies were going through. Already blaming myself for them not surviving. Blaming myself for what their lives would be like if they did somehow survive. What did I do to cause them to be conjoined? Did I eat something that I wasn't supposed to? Was God punishing me somehow? There was no one that was going to tell me that this wasn't my fault. No one could tell me that I wasn't to blame for all of this.

If I'm being honest, I sometimes still think about what I could have done that caused the girls to be conjoined. The truth is conjoined twins occur when the egg doesn't split completely. Depending on what you read, statistics will vary. The ones that I paid attention to is that conjoined twins occur in about 1 in every 200,000 births. Some statistics show that the survival rate after birth is between 5-25%.

13

I would spend hours and hours looking at articles about conjoined twins. I would search for any success story that would give me just an ounce of hope. There aren't many of those stories though. To put it into even more perspective, our twins were only the third set of conjoined twins born at Children's Hospital in Oklahoma City, since the 1980's.

I was obsessed with reading every story, every statistic, every outcome. I really would love to tell you that I was the person that hoped everything would be ok and that I knew in my heart that the twins would survive, but I wasn't. I envied my family that was pregnant. I envied my friends that were pregnant. I envied strangers that were pregnant. I envied anyone that had or would have children. I was in such a dark place that I wasn't sure that I would ever see light again. I didn't even like leaving my house because I didn't want to see a pregnant woman. I didn't want to be around children, at all. How does one really handle feeling like that? How could I be so resentful? Why did I feel like I was just an inch away from hating people that were happy? How could I not hate myself for feeling that way? I was always thinking about what could happen. I've heard before, why rehearse a tragedy, but that's exactly what I was doing. I was trying to prepare myself on how I would survive losing my babies. I wanted so badly to be able to enjoy my pregnancy, but the truth was that it was the absolute darkest time of my life.

For me, growing up and having children was always part of the plan. I couldn't wait to be a mom. I would dream about what life would be like having kids of my own. What their personalities would be like, what they would be when they grew up. I imagined all the good things that having children would bring. I suppose I was very naive about the whole thing really. You never really think about all the scary things that can happen. I mean, who would want to think that way anyway? I just assumed that everything would come easily and there wouldn't be any issues when I got pregnant. I knew that other people had complications with their pregnancies, but surely that wouldn't be me. It always happens to other people; it would never happen to me. The complications were a reality now. My reality was that this pregnancy was scary and not the one that I had planned for.

Some families with children facing medical complexities seek second, third, or even fourth opinions. We were so blessed to have an amazing medical team. Each tech, nurse, doctor and surgeon made us feel like such a priority. They wanted our babies to live and to thrive just as much as we did. So many people that we never even met played such a big role in our story. The maintenance men built a special bed for our twins in case the way they were positioned didn't allow them to lay in a typical bed. There were so many that would rehearse the delivery and separation surgery to make sure they were prepared to do their absolute best. They had two dolls, simulating how the twins were positioned in my tummy, that they used to practice their care with. They even went as far as telling us that they would have an elevator blocked off so that it would be available for when they were taking the twins from delivery to the NICU. Knowing that we had such a great team behind us was something that gave us an ounce of hope, and sometimes that ounce of hope would be the only thing getting me through the day.

The days seemed to be so long. I know for certain that I wasn't the only one hurting and scared of what would happen to our babies. However, when you're the mom, you don't get a break. Your growing belly, those random kicks, the morning sickness, they're all constant reminders that you're pregnant. I didn't have anything else to focus on. I didn't have other children to keep me busy. I wasn't working. I didn't have anything that could give me just a little bit of a distraction. I mentioned earlier that I like to be in control in just about every single way. I spent my days feeling out of control. I wasn't in control of how I was feeling: I wasn't in control of my grief, my anger, my jealousy. I wasn't in control of what was happening to our babies and I spent every single day feeling helpless.

As the date for their arrival was getting closer and closer, my anxiety and worry seemed to grow even more. I began realizing that they very well may make it to delivery. That was one major hurdle that we were about to jump over. My anxiety and worries were now shifting to whether or not they would be able to be separated. If they were able to be separated would they live through the surgery? What would life be like for them if they did live through it? My mom did something special for David and me during the last two weeks of my pregnancy. Every day we would get to open a single gift. Each day the gift was a cross. Those crosses reminded us that God is in control. Even though, I doubted Him so much, He had a plan. He was going to use our story for a purpose. My Mom wanted us to remember that. Those fourteen crosses are still hung on our wall.

14

Remember when I said that the babies were in an X shape. Read that as...there was no way that they were going to come out naturally. So, our c-section date was scheduled for July 7. I thought it was a good day, I always wanted a summer birthday as a kid and 7 is my favorite number. On the 4th of July, while I was at my dad's house, I was tired. More tired than I usually was. I could barely keep my eyes open. My bonus mom told me that she thought that I may be in labor. My stomach was as hard as a rock too. Nothing too crazy happened the rest of the night though. The next day, David and I spent the day together. I remember that I requested a cheeseburger that evening, so after we got one, we headed back home.

Later that evening I started feeling pretty strong contractions. I called my parents, and they came over (we were living in our condo then). They agreed that it was time to go to the hospital. I couldn't leave before my toenails were painted though. I realize that it should have been done way earlier but couldn't do much about it at that point. My dad was pacing back and forth, shaking his head, while my mom painted my toenails. Once she was finished it was time to load up in the car and get to the hospital.

Once we got there and checked in, the pain was almost more than I could handle. Throughout my pregnancy, I knew that I would be having a caesarean, so the thought of having actual labor pains, never even crossed my mind. I kept waiting for some relief, but it never seemed to come. At one point, I told the nurse that I wanted to go to the bathroom. She was reluctant to let me go but I did and passed out in the smallest bathroom you could imagine. My mom tried to wake me up as she was yelling for help. It was a weird sensation, it's almost like I could see things, but the world was standing still. I ended up passing out around 19 more times those next couple of days. There was nothing medically wrong with me at all. I think that my body had reached its breaking point. I did what I could to get our babies to that day alive, and my body was telling me that it had finally had enough.

My OB and her attending were able to make it for the delivery. I went back to the OR in the early morning of July 06. They say that I gave a thumbs up when I went back. I guess the pain was finally controlled and I was feeling pretty good because I don't really remember that at all. I remember sitting on the cold table waiting for the injection in my back. There were around 20 medical professionals in the room that in one way or another would help bring these babies into the world.

I'm sure I have mentioned it several times throughout this story, but the amount of supportive people in my life is overwhelming. My family and friends were getting up in the middle of the night to be there for the birth of the twins. They even brought lawn chairs and parked themselves in the waiting room as they waited for them to arrive. It's a good thing too because if they hadn't brought those lawn chairs, there wouldn't have been enough chairs for all of them. My sweet friend, Kim, prayed with those that were there. Another sweet friend, Rachel, shared that as they were all joined in prayer, there was an unexplainable peace that washed over them in that moment. To have that many people who love and support our family, be there during such a difficult time, was such a blessing.

15

On July 06, at 3:19am, Baby A hit the air of this world and immediately at 3:20am Baby B followed. People often ask which one is older, considering they were born conjoined and it makes sense that they would enter the world at the same time. However, at that point they were still in an X shape and Baby A was on top. I don't remember them crying when they came out, but I've read in the medical notes that there was crying. I was only able to see them for half a second as they wheeled them by me on their way to the NICU. I remember noticing that they were laying side by side as they went by. The medication had my brain in a fog, and I wasn't at full capacity so I couldn't remember why them laying side by side was good, I just knew that it was. The reason that it was good though, was because they were not laying on top of each other, with the possibility of the one on top suffocating the one on the bottom. They had the special bed in place if need be, but the fact that they didn't have to use it was amazing. The other reason it was good was because giving them oxygen and/or anesthesia would be much easier. David followed the twins up to the NICU where they would get checked out. I clearly stayed behind while they finished putting me back together. Funny story: I really loved my delivery nurse; she was the same one that I had the night before. I remember after David left with the twins, wanting her to sit with me. The attending OB came from around the curtain and said, she's busy. She was on the other side of the curtain doing her job, so the anesthesiologist kept me company instead.

Once I made it back to my room, David Facetimed us. He showed us the twins and they were beautiful. We were all asking him if they were boys or girls. He told us that they were girls, and I was over the moon. They told me that I had to be able to walk before I could go and see them. I think I willed myself to walk because I was able to get to them pretty quickly, I think that has to do with being a mom. Moms have superpowers.

It was surreal seeing Hartlyn and Everlee for the first time outside my tummy. Usually, moms are able to hold their child/children after they're delivered. That wasn't the case for me though. I didn't get to hold them right after delivery or even when they made it to the NICU. I actually didn't get to hold them until around day four and it was hard.

Finally being able to give them a name was amazing. I've told you several times throughout this book, how much I love names. Now, I want to share with you why we chose the names we did. Lisa, one of my favorite bosses of mine, was such a steady encourager throughout my pregnancy. When Lisa found out that the twins were conjoined, she would always refer to them as blessed babies who have a purpose and will bless so many around them. She had sent me the name Hartlyn several months before. I loved that name and added it to my very short list that I had going. While I was talking to my mom one day, we were thinking about how each time I got to hear their heartbeats, I would be able to make it through the day just a little easier. How perfect would that name be for one of them. Symbolizing those perfect and strong heartbeats that we heard.

I chose Hartlyn for Baby A and her middle name Amira, for a miracle. David chose Everlee (I told you he was good) for Baby B and she is forever our miracle. Her middle name is Ilya for I love you always. Their names have such powerful meanings. Their names have a story, just like I hoped they would. Although, I loved the boy names that we had picked, I was so excited that they were girls and that we had given them such meaningful names.

16

Despite all the statistics that we had been reading for the past several months, they were here. They were alive and they were beautiful. It was the day after they were born that we started to meet with the medical team that would be performing their separation. We met with Dr. Kropp and Dr. Palmer along with Emily, the social worker for the urology team. I remember our family sitting around a table in a room and Dr. Kropp saying things, but it seemed to just go over my head. I could hardly make sense of anything because I was still in so much pain and taking whatever pain medication they would give me. There were a few things that stood out, and one of those things was that they needed to be separated immediately. Initially, we thought that we would have at least a month before the separation surgery would be attempted. However, the twins were born with a life-threatening condition and separation needed to happen immediately. In fact, it was so urgent that another family whose child was scheduled for surgery, graciously gave us their child's surgery date, so that our babies could receive their emergency surgery the following day.

I didn't have too long to process that our babies would be heading into surgery at just two days old. I wasn't even discharged from the hospital yet. I'm certain that I could have had years to try to prepare to hand over my babies to a medical team, with the possibility of them not surviving, and it wouldn't have been any easier.

We spent the next day with them in their room. Even though I was so happy to have them here, I felt like I couldn't allow myself to fully let go of the fear I had that they would be taken from us.

The surgery was scheduled for the morning of July 8th. Our parents were with us as we prayed over them, asking God to allow them to come back to us. I was wheeled down to the holding room. Once I got to the holding room, Dr. Letton, was waiting for me with a consent to treat form. That was the hardest time that I ever had to write my name. When I put my name on that piece of paper, I was legally allowing the surgeons to take our babies to the operating room for a life or death surgery. I knew that for them to survive they had to have the surgery, but I also knew that if they didn't survive, it was my name on that consent form.

We didn't really know how long the surgery would last. We still didn't know exactly what they shared and what their outcome would be. They told us that a nurse would call every hour to give us updates. David and I were together in a room, while our family and friends waited in the waiting room.

I don't even think that David and I spoke while we waited. I was trying not to have a panic attack as I waited for the first update from the nurse. She did call at the one-hour mark and told us that the surgery had begun. She would call two more times to let us know that things were going well. As we got near hour four of the surgery, Dr. Letton walked in. He came into the room and I couldn't tell anything by his expression. My heart dropped because we had never gotten the final update telling us that the surgery was complete. He walked across the room and sat down in a chair. He looked at us and told us that they were separated, in recovery and doing great. He was rather calm and I'm sure exhausted, as the rest of the medical team probably was. After he said those words that we had been waiting to hear, David and I broke down. We were so overwhelmed with emotion. I remember David just putting his face in his hands and this time crying happy tears. Something that I didn't believe would happen, did. God answered our prayers and we had two separate babies.

17

Hartlyn and Everlee shared their colon and bladder, as well as one main artery. During the surgery, they split their colon and bladder, allowing each of the girls to have half of each organ. It still blows my mind all that they were able to do for them during that surgery. After surgery, they were taken to the NICU where they would begin their recovery. When we finally got to see them, it was even more surreal seeing them in separate beds than it was seeing them conjoined. I spent so many months thinking that there was no way that they would be able to be separated, if they did survive, that I was having a hard time processing it.

During the surgery, they used colored tape to keep everything separated. Hartlyn had orange tape around all of her wires and equipment and Everlee had blue. To this day when I see those colors together, I'm taken back to those days that we were in the hospital.

Would you believe me if I told you that they only spent a total of 19 days in the hospital? That's including being born, separated and recovering. I'd probably find it hard to believe if I wasn't there to witness it. The time they spent in the hospital, they received incredible care by the entire medical team. I felt as if God gave me the very best people to take care of our daughters and that He specifically chose them to be a part of our story. The nurses and doctors always stayed on top of their care. They made sure that we knew exactly what was going on and answered the millions of questions I had. It's amazing to think about what those 3lb and 4lb babies endured and what they overcame in such a short amount of time.

18

Because I didn't know and didn't think that they would survive, we didn't have anything prepared for them to go home. We didn't have a nursery set up, we didn't have clothes and we didn't even have car seats. David and I were frantic to get everything we needed so that when they were able to go home, we were ready. Thanks to our family, they helped us get all that we needed and when it was time to go home, we were ready.

We got to go home on that 19th day, and it was the best feeling in the world. They had the cutest going home dresses that my mom picked out, and we were welcomed home with signs and balloons from our family. They were already very loved by everyone and it showed so much.

David is from Macomb, a small town in Oklahoma. I've lived in Oklahoma my entire life and had never heard of it until I met him. It's your typical small town where everyone knows everyone and most everyone would do anything for anyone else. After the girls had made it home, some very special people from his hometown wanted to do a benefit for our family. Kathy, along with her family, found so many people that were happy to help in whatever way they could. She gathered up so many that were happy to help in whatever way they could. They raised money for us to help in whatever way we needed. They had a cookout, auction, and made t-shirts. They raised so much awareness that it even made the local news. The outpouring of love from that small town is something that our family will never forget. There are far too many people to name specifically, but I hope that they know just how much our family was blessed by all that they did for us.

The first several months I had a lot of help. David was working a pretty crazy work schedule so on the days that he would be gone overnight, one of my parents would stay with me. It was a big adjustment trying to take care of two babies. I was exhausted to say the least. I'm still not certain that I've caught up on all the sleep that I missed out on either.

I wanted to celebrate them all the time. So much so that we had a party around the 6th of every month. The parties were complete with family, friends, and cupcakes. It was very important to me that I made up for all the times that I didn't celebrate them while I was pregnant. I feel like there were many things that I was too depressed to enjoy and I wanted to make up for lost time.

I think part of the reason that I wanted to celebrate them each month was because deep down I still didn't believe that they were here or that they were as healthy as they were. I spent months anticipating them not surviving, (yes, I know how horrible that sounds), so I wanted a reminder that they were here, that they made it home.

We weren't home too long before we learned that Hartlyn had hip dysplasia. I'm clearly no medical professional but basically hip dysplasia is when the hip socket doesn't fully cover the ball portion of the thighbone. So, when she was just a couple months old, she got a cast on her leg. It was a soft cast and was changed every couple of weeks. I would draw on them, just to make them a little bit easier to look at. It was hard to see her in those but really, it was what she needed, and she seemed to tolerate them well. Thankfully, she didn't need any other medical intervention, like physical therapy or surgery.

We would go to the usual baby checkups where the twins would just do their thing and show us all how strong they truly are. They were happy, healthy and thriving, and I was so grateful that God allowed us to keep them here with us.

Their main surgeon and doctor that we still follow up with to this day is Dr. Kropp who we saw when they were first born and one of the four that separated them. He told us early on after they were born that they would need to have an invasive reconstructive surgery and that they could have it as early as a year old. They would need to have their pelvis broken and rods placed in them so that they could move their anatomy around, which would allow them to be as healthy as possible as they grow.

I spent most of the days during their first year of life thinking about the surgery that I knew they would be having one day. I felt like we made it through such a hard and unknown time, and now I was spending days dreading having to hand them off to surgeons again for the second time in their short little lives. I just wanted to enjoy my girls without fear of what the future would bring but it was so hard. Don't get me wrong, I loved the days that I had with them and was so thankful for the time that I never thought I'd have. But knowing the day would come where we were once again in the hospital, watching our babies go through so much, was difficult.

Their first year was spent making many memories and accomplishing every milestone that they were supposed to. From them rolling over, to sitting up on their own, then walking, and all the things that I never even allowed myself to dream about after I found out that they were conjoined. I was overwhelmed by all their "firsts" because it was happening in real life. They were doing things that statistics told me probably would never happen and I was soaking it all in. Watching their personalities develop was such a joy.

Once they turned one, we started really thinking about when their next surgery would take place. Dr. Kropp, Dr. Palmer and Emily all moved to Cook Children's Hospital in Fort Worth, Texas by the time that the twins turned one. Because most of the reconstructive surgery would be with the urology team, we knew that we would be traveling to have them do the surgery. This surgery would be an extensive recovery and would require us to stay in Texas for an extended amount of time. We had to figure out the logistics of how it would be possible for us to stay close to the hospital considering we had our house and all the bills to go with it back in Oklahoma.

Something else really cool happened when they turned one. The hospital decided to have a get together with all of those from their medical team that could attend. I can hardly describe how amazing it was to see the girls reunited with those that took such great care of them. To show them how Hartlyn and Everlee were thriving and so full of life, is something that I'll never forget. I hope that when they saw how happy and healthy the girls were, that they know just how big of a role they each played in making that happen.

After a lot of thought, we decided that the girls would have the surgery when they were around 2.5 years old. It was exhausting trying to figure out how we were going to balance everything considering that we would more than likely be in Texas for a few months. Once again, our family, friends and the town of Macomb, rallied around our little family. A really nice guy, Brad, organized a fundraiser for us too. They raised money that would help us stay in Texas for the length of the twins' recovery. This was amazing because it also allowed David to take off work and be there with us the entire time. There is so much that can worry a parent who has a child or children with medical complexities. Not having to worry about the financial aspect of it all was a huge relief.

Remember when I said that my parents all got along? I am about to blow some minds with this part of the story. Because of how many of us wanted to be there with the girls as much as we possibly could be, we had to get an apartment. Most children's hospitals have places where families can stay but when you are blessed with a family like ours, you need more room. My cousin in Texas helped us to find a two-bedroom apartment just about two blocks from where Hartlyn and Everlee would be having their surgery. One day, my dad, mom and I traveled down to Fort Worth to check out the apartment and sign the lease. I will give you all a second to take that in. Yes, all four of my parents would at some point or another be staying in the same two-bedroom apartment with David and me. David's parents and even some of our siblings would stay there some of the time during our few months in the apartment. My mom was retired from teaching and my dad had also retired by this point. They would be there the entire time and my bonus mom and bonus dad would be with us when they didn't have to work.

We packed up what we would be needing for the next few months and made our way down to Texas on October 15, 2016. I remember that day specifically because it's David's and my anniversary, just in case you want to send us a card. It was like we were just starting out and getting our first place. My dad and bonus mom bought all sorts of things to take with us. We even got new dishes and living room furniture (that we still use to this day). We got settled into the apartment once we got down there and it felt good to feel like we had a home away from home.

The next day, we headed to the hospital to meet with the surgeons that would be performing their reconstructive surgery. We pulled up to the hospital, and I had gotten one of the twins out of their car seat. It had been raining, and right after I handed her off to whichever family member was beside me, I fell on the concrete. When I say I fell, I mean I fell hard. It was a mixture of pain followed by tears of humiliation. I was so embarrassed. Our first appointment that day was with Dr. Gray, the orthopedic pediatric surgeon. When he walked into the room, I was propped up on the table with ice on my knee. He looked at me and asked if I was the patient. We all had a good laugh about how clumsy I am. I knew that I would like him from that moment because having a sense of humor in such a scary time, makes it just a bit easier, even if it's just for a minute.

The twins would each have two days' worth of surgery. Hartlyn would have one surgery October 17th, then they would both be in the OR the 18th, and Everlee would have her second day of surgery on the 19th.

The night of Hartlyn's first surgery was the first night that the twins had ever spent the night apart. Before that night, they had spent every night of their lives in the same room, right next to each other. I know they were young, but I would imagine they missed each other and wondered why they weren't together. They Facetimed with each other and that was at least better than nothing.

This go round was different for me than their separation surgery. I was coherent and much more aware of what was going on. When the twins had their separation surgery, I wasn't even discharged from the hospital yet, was on pain medication, and had a hard time processing everything that was going on. This time though, I was present, and my anxiety was incredibly high. I knew this wasn't a life-or-death scenario like it was when they were two days old, but it's still never easy when your children have to endure something like surgery. It wasn't just one surgery but two, and those surgeries would be incredibly painful and came with an extensive recovery time.

Hartlyn's first surgery lasted around four hours and Everlee's first surgery was about eight hours. During their first surgery is when they broke their pelvises. It would allow for the organs that needed to be moved around, to stay where they needed to once they healed. It's hard to understand and even harder to explain, but as painful as that sounds, they absolutely had to do it. They would each have "external fixators" and they looked just as painful as they sound. It looked like spikes coming out of them and that's what was holding their bones in place so that when they healed, they would be in the correct place.

Their second surgery was with the urologists, Dr. Kropp and Dr. Palmer. They did reconstruction on some of their organs and moved other organs around. Hartlyn's surgery lasted for fourteen hours and Everlee's lasted for eight.

After Hartlyn finished her second surgery, her epidural that they had put in for pain got a kink in it and stopped working. It was around midnight, and I had gone back to the apartment with my mom to get some rest while David stayed with the twins. The doctors and nurses tried for hours to get her pain under control, but nothing seemed to work. Finally, they decided to put her back under anesthesia so that they could put in another epidural. David witnessed more of this than I did, and I know that it's something he will never forget. Seeing your child in that amount of pain is something that sticks with you.

The twins were in the pediatric intensive care unit for almost a week before they were able to go to a regular room. When they got to their new room, they were finally able to be together again. It was nice to have them both in the same place. It was heartbreaking that we weren't able to be in two places at one time, so I was thankful that we had made it to this point. Hartlyn would say, "Sissy" and show us her IV's. She would also say, "better." I'd wonder what was going through their minds and really hoped that they wouldn't remember all of the pain that they were in.

A week after their surgery, we were able to put them in wagons and take them around the hospital and we even got to venture outside. They each had a wagon and would hold hands while they were side by side. It was nice to be able to take them out of their rooms for a change in scenery as we went on walks throughout the day. It made the days seem not so long.

On October 27th, we were discharged from the hospital. To have those big surgeries out of the way was such a relief. I had worried and anticipated those for so long and it felt like a weight had been lifted, knowing that that part of the story was behind us. The girls had an amazing medical team, but it was nice to finally have them in our "temporary home" so that they could rest without so much interruption.

19

Being discharged was a bit tricky. The hardware that they had around their pelvises made it where they weren't able to fit in a car seat. So, because the apartment was within walking distance from the hospital, they were discharged in those cool wagons that we got to take them around the hospital in. We bundled them up, put them in their special wagons, and we walked a couple of blocks to our apartment. We weren't going to let anything stop us from getting to the next stage of recovery.

Remember when I described the metal thing that looked like it had spikes coming out of it? They still had those and would have to have them for a total of six weeks. They were both prescribed pain medication to help with the pain. I don't know if it was Hartlyn's experience with the failed epidural or what, but we couldn't get her to take the pain medication. We tried everything, but she wasn't having it. We couldn't even get her to take Tylenol or Motrin really. Can you imagine having pins in your bones, unable to really move, and not have any pain medication?

Not only did the girls have to wear those medieval devices, but we had to change the dressings around them. It was hard on my heart doing it because I know that it was painful for them. I was adamant about it though, and even a tad controlling because I wanted to make sure that it was done the right way. I know how that makes me sound, and my husband and family were totally capable of doing it but, I just had to do it myself. I had to be the one to do it. I think it's a mother thing.

They were able to get the pins out a week earlier than we thought. The doctors said it was because of how well they were taken care of and how quickly their bodies healed. I also know how that makes me sound, like "go me" right? But I think that it's important for me to say that even though things can be hard for us when it comes to our children, we push through it because it's what's best for them and most likely what they need. So, when you deserve a pat on the back, give yourself one.

We spent Thanksgiving at the apartment. It was a little bit different not being home but having all four of my parents there, David and the twins, I couldn't have asked for much better. We cooked a great Thanksgiving meal in that tiny apartment kitchen, and we all sat around the table with so much to be thankful for.

The days would come and go. We were so happy to see them without that contraption on, but they still had a long way to go. They wouldn't be able to put any weight on their legs for another two weeks. After that two weeks, we would be able to help them start to walk again. We had decided to stay at the apartment until December 6th, which would be their final check-up post-surgery.

The two weeks passed, and we started working on teaching them to walk again. They would hold our hands and would take a few steps and then would crawl the rest of the way to get to where they wanted to go. I remember on the day that we first started working with them, they were cheering each other on and giving high-fives. Those days are ones that are etched in my mind. They were so brave, resilient, and strong. Those tiny girls were learning how to walk for a second time, and I was one proud Mama Bear.

We also started packing to go home on December 6th. We were so beyond ready to go back home and start a new chapter. It was almost surreal to think that we were finally able to go home. We loaded up the next day and headed back to Oklahoma. Once we got home, Hartlyn would say, “made it home” and those weren’t just simple words to me. Even as I am writing this now, I’m emotional because they did, they did make it back home. From the day that the doctors told us that this would be a huge, painful, long recovery surgery, I had worried about it. I had spent two years never too far away from thinking about what that surgery would be like for the girls. I was so thankful to have that behind us, and for the first time in a long time, I felt like I could breathe a bit easier.

On December 17th, Hartlyn started walking again and Everlee followed on December 28th. We were finally on our way to having them back to running all over the place and us trying to keep up. It was amazing knowing that just a few weeks earlier, they had their pelvises broken and weren’t really able to move for over 5 weeks. I’ve known since they were born that they were strong little girls, but this brought it to a whole new level. Here they were, walking and jumping again, just as if nothing happened.

20

So much life has happened since they were born. So many things that I thought that they wouldn't be able to do or even be alive to do, they're doing. Before I became pregnant, I would always think about what my children would be like. Would they play an instrument or sports? Both? What would they be when they grew up? Once I found out about them being conjoined, I stopped wondering about all those things and just wondered if they would survive.

When they were able to start PreK, I was completely terrified. Not because they weren't healthy enough but because I would be handing off their care to someone else if they went to public school. I really went back and forth about what the right decision would be for them. It finally came down to this: I want Hartlyn and Everlee to know that they are capable of anything and everything that they want to do in life. I don't want them to feel like any differences that they have limit them in any way. They are strong, brave, resilient, beautiful girls and I never want them to think otherwise.

As a mother, you can often feel mom-shamed. I mean sure, there are mothers who we think (absolutely know) should not be mothers, you know the ones that for whatever reason are unable to care for their child or children but that's not what I'm referring to. There are two things that really and truly infuriate me. Those two things are conversations about breast feeding and the actual birth of the child/children. I would love for you to hear me out on this.

First off, let's talk about breastfeeding. I am super aware of all the benefits of breastfeeding. However, it's just not all that simple for some of us moms. For me personally, it was incredibly challenging. For one, I had two children to feed. The other major contributing factor is that I was so physically and mentally drained from my pregnancy and them actually being here, that a lot of times, I would go home and rest at night. I applaud all the parents that can be at the bedside nonstop and never leave, but to be honest, that's not me. I will get to where I can no longer function and I promise, it's not fun to witness. Thankfully, as I have mentioned several other times, my family is amazing. My mom would take the night shift and my bonus mom would be there in the morning.

David and I would go back to the hospital in the late morning and stay until night. The twins were never alone. All of that to say this: I did try breastfeeding. I would set alarms but most of the time would be so tired that I just couldn't make myself get up to pump. Of course, there was one doctor who really wanted to make sure that I knew just how much better breast milk was for the twins. After I told her that I just could not keep up, she wanted us to use donated breastmilk. I think that is so awesome that there are moms that donate their breast milk, and we did use the milk bank while we were in the NICU, but we weren't able to go home on donated milk. We weren't looking at a long hospital stay so I feel like the whole conversation was almost pointless. There should not be any conversations regarding the best way to feed your child when clearly it's not be your "typical" birth. As long as the pros are known, mothers should be able to feel that they are able to choose the feeding option that works best for them and their child. I think we should all be able to agree that fed is best. The reasons that a baby is formula fed instead of breastfed may be more complicated than it seems.

The other thing that truly OFFENDS me is when people say that having a c-section is the easy way out or even worse that it's not really giving birth, it's just surgery. I'm going to take this time again to mention that the twins were in the shape of an X inside my tummy. There is absolutely no way on earth that they would have come out "naturally", they wouldn't have survived. Even before I found out they were conjoined, I was told that it's suggested in most cases that a c-section is planned for twins, even without any concerns found during pregnancy. With my lack of pain tolerance, even when I thought I was just having one baby, I had decided that I would probably have a c-section because I was too scared to do it the other way. There is nothing easy about having a c-section in case you didn't know. No matter the way a child comes into this world, it's a beautiful thing.

One thing that has been especially important to me is making sure that Hartlyn and Everlee love themselves, however their bodies may be. Sharing their colon and bladder means that they are going to have differences. They are different from their family, their friends and most everyone else that they meet. While they are young, I can mostly shield them from the outside world. With that said though, I am teaching them to know just how special they are. I am teaching them that God made them just the way He wanted to. I wish I could say that everyone they meet who finds out about their differences, will be kind, but that's just not realistic. So as a mom, who desperately wants her children to always love themselves, please remember to be kind to everyone. Teach your kids to be kind. My girls deserve to be accepted by everyone.

David and I have talked over the years about having at least one more child. I could never explain what my biggest fear about having another child was though. The odds of us having conjoined twins again is slim to none, but the fear and the worry is hard to ignore. Being in the world of medical complexities with my own children, I feel like I am more aware of all the scary things that can happen than I used to be.

I also feel like the twins and I have a bond that I don't want to ever lose. I'm sure there are other moms that feel that way after they've had their first baby. Wondering, how am I going to love another baby as much as I love my first (first two in my case)? I feel that way too, but also on a deeper level. In a sense, I feel like it was the twins and me against the world. It was us (mostly them), fighting to get here and stay here. Something that I would tell the twins while I was pregnant was that I need them to fight to be here just as hard as I was fighting for them. It's kind of hard to think about that though because I really felt like I was barely existing while I was pregnant. I don't want to feel like the bond I would have with any future child is less significant than the bond that I have with the twins.

After praying and searching my heart for my true feelings, I came to the conclusion that I was just scared of what could happen to my baby whether it was while I was pregnant or after. I still, to this day, suffer from PTSD. I know that you usually don't hear about PTSD caused by pregnancy, but I assure you that it is real and something I still battle to this day. To be honest, I can hardly watch gender reveal parties and still have a hard time going to baby showers. If I'm being absolutely transparent, I still have a hard time when I see pregnant women. I am very aware of how that sounds, and I really wish that I didn't feel the way I do but I'm putting it all out there. It's a back and forth feeling because on one hand, I am jealous of the "normal" pregnancy that they may have but I also know that if I didn't have the journey that I did, I wouldn't have Hartlyn and

Everlee. That's a life that I don't want to even imagine.

21

I have had therapists off and on throughout my life. I have had them to help with depression, anxiety, anger, OCD: the whole kit and caboodle that is my mental health. I think it's so important for people to know that you don't have to have severe mental health issues to speak with a therapist. I have a therapist that I speak to every month. I talk to her about everything under the sun and the last few meetings we have been discussing my anxieties about having more children. I told her all the things I am telling you and her response to me was that I cannot make decisions based out of fear. I can't let fear dictate my life and what I get out of it.

No matter what hardships come my way, I have to be strong for the girls. They need to know that they can face anything in life and be okay. I need to be an example for them, and that means I have to face my fears no matter how legitimate those fears are.

There was a time in my life when I couldn't even make it through a breakup without being depressed and thinking that the world was ending. Since having Hartlyn and Everlee, I have made it through some of the hardest times of my life so far and there is no doubt in my mind that it's because of them. I look at them and think of all the things they had to go through just to get to today. They have been through more in their short lives, than most of us will experience in a lifetime.

Do you ever think to yourself, if I could just let my younger self know…?

I'd love to go back in time and tell myself so many things. For one, I would tell my younger self that life is full of unknowns and things that are out of your control. To have faith that things are going to work out the way that they are meant and intended to. It may not be in the way that you want it or think that it should be, but there is a reason and usually there is always a silver lining.

I would tell myself that happiness is what you make it. It doesn't depend on if you go to college, or in my case, finish college. It doesn't depend on when or if you get married. It doesn't depend on what your house looks like or the car you drive. It doesn't matter how much you have in the bank or if you keep up with the Joneses. None of those are ways to fill your heart. Your heart is filled by love, kindness, joy, hope and gratefulness. Those are things that will make you genuinely happy. I searched for happiness in so many wrong places, but I am here to tell you that having the girls in my life has opened up my eyes on what being happy really means.

I would tell myself that people are people and doctors are people too. I spent so many weeks and months focusing on every bad statistic out there regarding conjoined twins. I focused too heavily on what the first specialist told us and not enough into what God had planned for me. No matter what His plan was, I should have accepted it and known that whatever was going to happen would and it would be because that's the way it was meant to happen.

I would tell myself that I am capable. From being someone who wasn't really allowed to teach her younger siblings their body parts when they were learning them (so confusing), to being the mother of twin girls that each have their own unique anatomy to learn. When I say unique, I mean having our doctor draw pictures so that I may have somewhat of a clue as to what was going on with their bodies. I am capable of being their Mom.

I have so much hope for Hartlyn and Everlee's future. More than anything, I want them to always know how special they are. I want them to know in their hearts that they were put on this Earth for a purpose and that God has big things planned for them. They have the ability to inspire so many people and I pray that they do. I pray that they want to do that, that they want to share their story and their outlook on the world. I think that a lot of people could learn something from them and the amazing journey that they've had and will have for the rest of their lives.

The world can be a scary place. There are so many things that can "go wrong". We live with so many unknowns that we could drive ourselves crazy with all of the what-ifs. That's exactly what I did while I was pregnant, and I still do that today to an extent. The truth, though, is that we can miss out on so much life if we are waiting for the worst to happen.

The twins still have a major surgery to get through within the next year or two. It is pretty extensive with a long road to recovery. I could dwell on that, like I did while I was pregnant or while I was waiting for their second surgery when they were two years old, or I could choose to live in the here and now. I could choose to be happy that they have so much life that they get to live in between surgeries and doctors' appointments. They are happy, healthy and loving life.

22

If you know me, then you may know that I happen to thoroughly enjoy 90's country music. A big part of 90's country music was a guy with a big name from none other than the state of Oklahoma. There is a song that I often think about called, Unanswered Prayers. Have you ever really thanked God for some of your unanswered prayers? There was a time in my life when I prayed that an ex-boyfriend and I wouldn't break up. Years later, I prayed that my ex-husband and I wouldn't go through with our divorce. There was also a time, not too many years ago, that I prayed to God that if life was going to be too hard for our babies, to take them before they came into this world. Where would I be if God had answered all of those prayers in the way that I was praying He would? I would not have met the man that's the love of my life, I wouldn't have had the continuous up and down journey of motherhood and I most certainly wouldn't have been blessed with these two miracles that call me Mom. Sometimes the best gift God can give us, is unanswered prayers.

Hartlyn and Everlee made me a better person. They opened my heart more than I thought that anyone would be able to. It's not always easy and I've got a lot of room for improvement, but I am so blessed to be their mom. God gave me the biggest challenge with the greatest reward when He gave me them. I hope they always know how much I love them.

I didn't write our story to gain sympathy or pity. Ever since I've had the girls, I struggle when people say, "I'm so sorry" or "there's no way that I could handle all of that". The truth is that our journey was hard, incredibly hard. The reason that I wrote this story is because I want there to be stories out there that have happy endings. I want to tell a story that gives others the hope that I was desperately searching for. I want Hartlyn and Everlee to be an inspiration to every last person on Earth and to see that anything is possible.

I want people that hear devastating news to know that there is always hope. Even when things don't go as planned, it's ok to be angry and sad. It's a part of your story and there's no shame in that. Eventually though, find your joy again. Find a way to help others going through a similar journey. There's strength in numbers.

It would be absolutely impossible for me to thank everyone that has been in our story, but I would at least like to do an overall thank you because it would be wrong not to.

For those that had a role in being a part of our medical team, thank you. Thank you for your knowledge, your care, your dedication, and for bringing our girls into the world. Thank you to the ones that are still a part of the twins' care. We have trusted you from the beginning and always will.

For David's hometown of Macomb, OK: Thank you all for loving and supporting our family through the years. The amount of love that you have shown us has been nothing less than amazing. With your help, we were able to be together as a family during such a difficult time. We will never be able to tell you just how much we appreciate you.

For the maintenance men at Children's Hospital: You all prepared for the arrival of our twins by making them a comfortable and safe place to rest and we are so grateful. Thank you for going above and beyond your job to make sure our babies were well taken care of.

To our family: I wouldn't have made it without you all. You were strong when I needed you most. You have been there with us every step of the way and God couldn't have given me a better family. Thank you for being the greatest. I love you more.

To my friends: Your encouraging words and prayers through my difficult time is something that I will never forget. Thank you for being a rock for me. I love you all.

To the doctors, statistics and all the other negativity I saw while I was pregnant: If it weren't for you, I wouldn't have a story to tell. I wouldn't have a reason to tell the world not to lose hope. Because of you, I have a mission to let the world know that anything is possible because our girls beat your odds.

Prayer Warriors: Thank you for the countless prayers you stormed Heaven with. The prayers were felt, and God heard them. Prayer is powerful and the twins are living proof.

To God: Without You, none of our story would be possible. You were there during both the hard and happy times. Even when my faith wavered, You were constant. Thank you for answering our prayers.

To my husband: Thank you for helping me create our precious girls. Thank you for celebrating our time on the mountaintops and sticking with me as we walked through the valleys. We have made it through what seemed impossible and we did it together. There's no one else that I would pick to be our girls' Daddy. The love you have for them and how proud of them you are, shines through. Your three ladies love you so very much.

Finally, to Hartlyn and Everlee: You two made me a mom. You are the double rainbow after my darkest storm. You both have shown me what God is truly capable of and are two of His greatest miracles. Live your life with your head held high and your heart open. You deserve all the good this world and Heaven has to offer. Being your Mom is the absolute honor of my life. I pray that you always know your worth and that you know that your dreams are achievable. You sweet girls have an amazing journey ahead of you, and I'm thankful for my front row seat. I love you both more than words could possibly say.

Notes from the Medical Team

The team was so beyond prepared that they even had the elevator blocked off for when the twins arrived and needed to make it to the NICU to begin their care.

Thoughts from our team:

First, when at Cook for the girl's bladder reconstructions, when they were done one day after the other, every nurse or staff that helped with the girls' care would ask me about how they were doing and check in on their recovery for weeks on end. For about a month after their surgeries, everywhere I went in the hospital and clinic, I would constantly be asked. The way the girls and your family impacted everyone they encountered during their journey in the hospital was not surprising to me, but special for sure.

Second, a cool memory for me, was when I unexpectedly ran into you and the girls in Dallas at the 3v3 basketball fundraiser. I recognized you quickly, but I almost didn't recognize the girls because they had grown up so much and were running around intermixed with all the other kids. It was so cool to see them. It was a combination of appreciating them as the normal kids that they are but special to know the journey they had been on. It was just any other day for them but for me to see them outside of the hospital/clinic was a special moment.

- Dr. Blake Palmer, M.D.

During my maternal fetal medicine training, I had the privilege of caring for Khalie during her high-risk pregnancy complicated by omphalopagus conjoined twins. As a fellow in the middle of Maternal Fetal Medicine training, it is a pregnancy I will never forget. We learn that conjoined twins are a rare subset of twins in which incomplete division occurs, resulting in varying degrees of fusion of the twins at the same anatomic site. They are so rare, that we think conjoined twins happen approximately 1 in 100,000 births.

I will never forget the first time viewing the ultrasound images of Khalie at 24 weeks, it was like watching two twins essentially dancing in the uterus at 90-degree angles to each other. For the next several weeks I watched as these twins grew and continued their beautiful little dance, and each week Khalie and the twins kept defying the odds. The strength and hope Khalie brought to each visit was both inspiring and humbling. This was not an easy pregnancy. The anxiety and the weight are not one I would wish on any of my patients, but Khalie took it one day at a time and for that reason alone she and these twins are a pregnancy I will never forget.

In the last couple weeks, we met several times as a medical team to practice and coordinate the delivery of these twin girls. However, much like many pregnancies, labor is unpredictable, and they decided to make their debut earlier than expected. Walking into the operating room, delivering and then finally meeting these little girls I was filled with immeasurable relief. Delivering these twins is an experience I will always remember. I will remember gently nudging one twin out and then carefully rotating to cradle and deliver the co-twin before handing them over to the waiting team of neonatologists.

In the end it could not have gone any better. In the days that followed, the successful separation of Hartlyn and Everlee, made everything worth it. To this day, I keep the picture Khalie gifted me of the twins on my desk, as it reminds me of the privilege of caring for women and their babies during some of the most vulnerable times of both woman and motherhood.

Dr. Asal Fathian, MD, MS, MHA, FACOG

Conjoined twins are a fascinating group of patients with variable presentations. The process is even more meaningful when our OU medical team provides care for a patient as wonderful as you. The type of your infants' connection (omphalopagus) influenced our planning, management, and kind of delivery. As such, your delivery required care from multiple specialists at OU. What I remember the most about our experiences was your realistic yet hopeful outlook of the care leading up to the delivery. It was no secret that your pregnancy's potential to end poorly was a real issue, yet you continued to maintain a positive outlook. As you recall, we carefully planned multiple meetings with the various specialists and organized a delivery simulation trying to anticipate your needs as well as the twins. When I received the call that you had presented to the L&D in labor, and we performed the cesarean delivery, it could not have gone any better. I know that the outcome was due to your positive attitude and the trust that you placed in our teams (MFM, NICU, and the Pediatric surgical subspecialties). Thank you for your trust my friend.

Dr. Marvin Williams, DO, FACOG
Professor, Section of Maternal-Fetal Medicine
Department of Obstetrics and Gynecology

"Dr. Kropp, you are never going to believe this! There is a set of conjoined twins that both have ***** and they are connected by their urinary bladders and bowel." This is what I was told by my urology resident team after the Perez twins were born. Now you can imagine my mind starting to calculate the odds of this happening. Both conditions occurring at the same time is a statistical "one in a trillion" occurrence. Immediately, I thought, "How am I going to solve this problem?" or simply how was I going to first separate the girls and then make it possible for both Hartlyn and Everlee to have the most normal life possible.

The first time I met with mom and dad and the extended family I was impressed with how they all were so committed to these girls. There was nothing that any one of them would not have given to help these girls. Hartlyn and Everlee were true miracles and the family recognized this fact.

The initial separation of the twins was performed by team members from Urology, General Surgery, Anesthesia, Neonatology and all of the ancillary services at Children's Hospital of Oklahoma. This initial separation was extremely successful. With stage one complete, I could focus on rebuilding these beautiful little babies over the next 10 years to live full and productive lives.

Well, this same thought is still with me every day. I have spent hundreds of hours thinking, evaluating, and drawing pictures about the girls' reconstructions and explaining to the family the risks and benefits of every step in the process. Khalie and the rest of the family with their unwavering faith in these girls, treating them with a "no different than any other child attitude" has provided the foundation for the girls' success.

Over the years, my greatest joy has been watching the girls open up to me and let me into their circle of trust. Oh sure, many times it involved bribery with Starbursts but over the last year I can feel that they truly trust me. Many thanks to Khalie, their mother, for always setting clear guidelines for the girls on what is appropriate behavior. Mom dad and all of the extended family have given the girls a solid foundation of love, support, structure and stability and this is the reason Hartlyn and Everlee are having such a wonderful childhood.

I have always felt blessed for the opportunity to care for Hartlyn and Everlee. They are now much more than just a statistical anomaly of a rare birth defect. They are a part of my family here at OKC Kids Urology. It continues to be my honor to care for these wonderful and delightful girls and to be part of their lives. It will be exciting to watch all of the other chapters in their lives unfold as they navigate through the rest of childhood into adulthood.

Dr. Bradley P. Kropp, MD, FACS, FAAP
Medical Director, OKC Kids Urology PLLC

I was very privileged to be a part of this wonderful journey this family endured. I was involved early in the post-surgical recovery and post-operative care provided. It was a once in a lifetime opportunity to be an integral part of the Pediatric Urology team that was involved in the complex reconstruction and management process for the conjoined twins.

I have been able to watch the girls grow and develop over the last 5 years. Our Pediatric Urology Team has been able to help give them a better quality of life in regard to their bladder and bowel health. We all went through some very challenging times as we worked together to get the twins' bladder and bowel management as optimal as it could be. The family showed such resilience as they learned about the girls' management and navigated through the healthcare system.

The twins are currently doing very well and are as healthy as can be. I look forward to the many more years ahead getting to provide care for them.

Jake Klein, MS, ARNP, CPNP
Director of Reconstructive Surgery and
Continence Specialist, OKC Kids Urology

I met Everlee and Hartlyn's family before I met them, introducing myself as the clinical social worker on the medical team. I remember learning that these girls had not only a large family, but a dedicated, tough, and committed family. During each of their surgeries their parents, grandparents, uncles and aunts waited outside the operating room providing support and love to one another.

After Everlee and Hartlyn's bladder closures, they could not fit in any kind of car seat because of the hardware on their pelvises, so we discharged them in their very own Radio Flyer Wagons. In the wagons, they looked like warriors having had fought a hard fight and being sent home to be comforted and convalesce in their own special rides.

Emily Haddad, LCSW

My favorite memory of the twins was their one-year-old birthday party at The Children's Hospital. Their return meant so much to the doctors and nurses who rarely get to see the children after surgery. There were smiles everywhere and you could see on the faces of the OR team how much it meant to have a family return to thank them and share in the joy of celebrating these beautiful girls. I believe their journey has inspired many people and I was blessed to be a small part of their first year here.

Travis Doussette
*helped our family tell our story
through the media

A portion of my medical notes:

"Today we discussed the management of Khalie's pregnancy. She has been previously counseled about the option of pregnancy termination, and she has opted to continue the pregnancy. She is aware that the risk for stillbirth is relatively high and that these events may be difficult to predict due to stillbirth's multifactorial nature. She is also aware that surgical separation can be quite complicated."

These days Hartlyn and Everlee are your typical 5-year-olds. It's funny to me just how different our IDENTICAL twins are. Hartlyn loves sharks, dinosaurs, and outer space. Everlee loves mermaids, unicorns, and rainbows. Hartlyn is a type A personality and quite a perfectionist, while Everlee is much more carefree and loves putting on a show. No matter how different they are, they are each other's best friend. They have their disagreements and get on each other's nerves, (I can't fathom what their teenage years will be like), but they always look out for each other. If one didn't eat their dinner and can't have a snack, the other won't have a snack in solidarity. If one is hurt or sad, they comfort each other and it would melt your heart. It's truly a blessing to witness the twin bond that they share. There is nothing in the world that could break it.

I talk to the girls a lot about their story. Even though they are so young, I've been honest with them about how scared I was when I was pregnant. I want them to know that it's ok to be scared and ask God a million questions when you don't understand what's going on or how something is going to turn out. Because of how open I've been with my own feelings, it allows them to feel safe sharing their feelings and emotions with me. Their perspective is so encouraging, and I learn from them every day.

God is always with us no matter what. When you get pushed down, get back up. I know in my heart that I can get through anything. I want our story to encourage people that need it.

Hartlyn Amira age 5

God helps us get through hard times. God is always by our side; He never leaves us. I want people to have hope and to be brave. I want them to have courage to get through rough days.

Everlee Ilya age 5

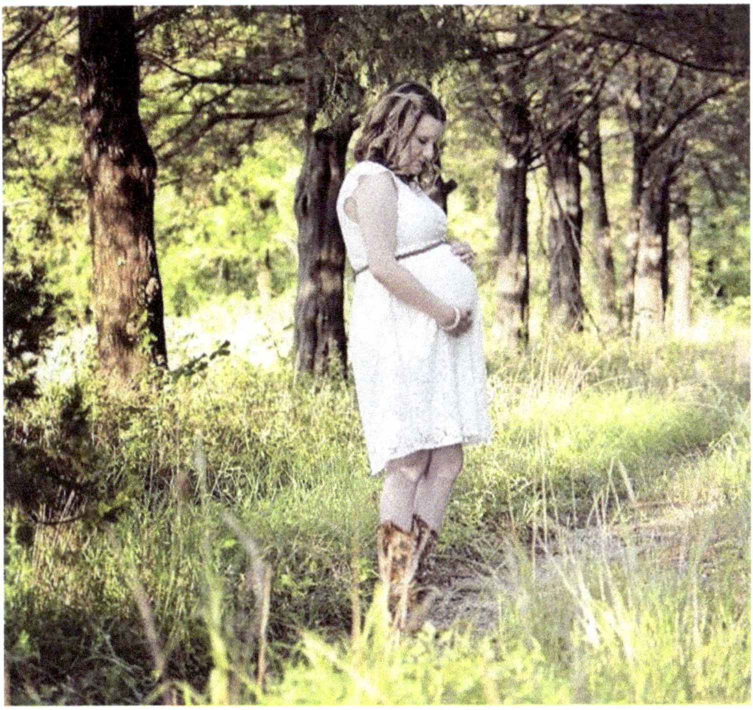

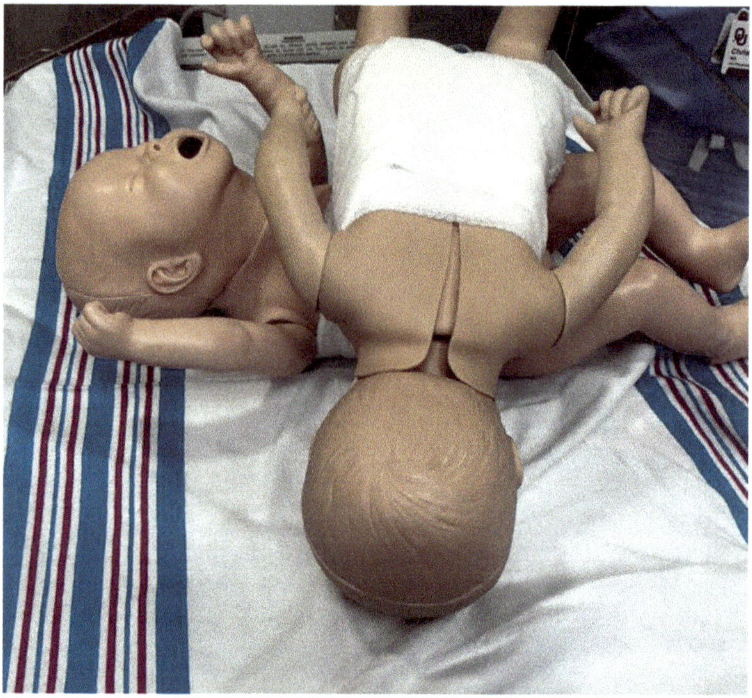

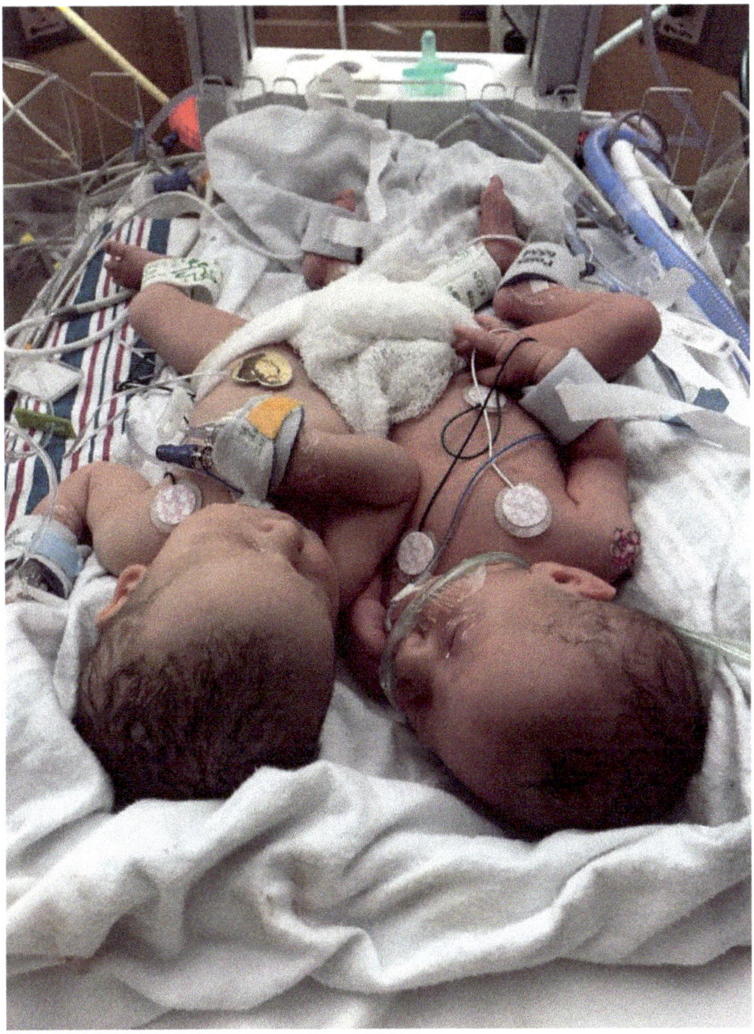

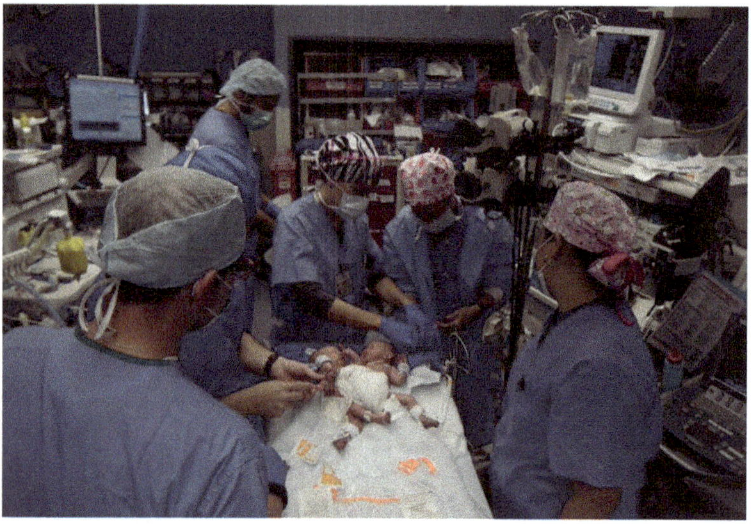

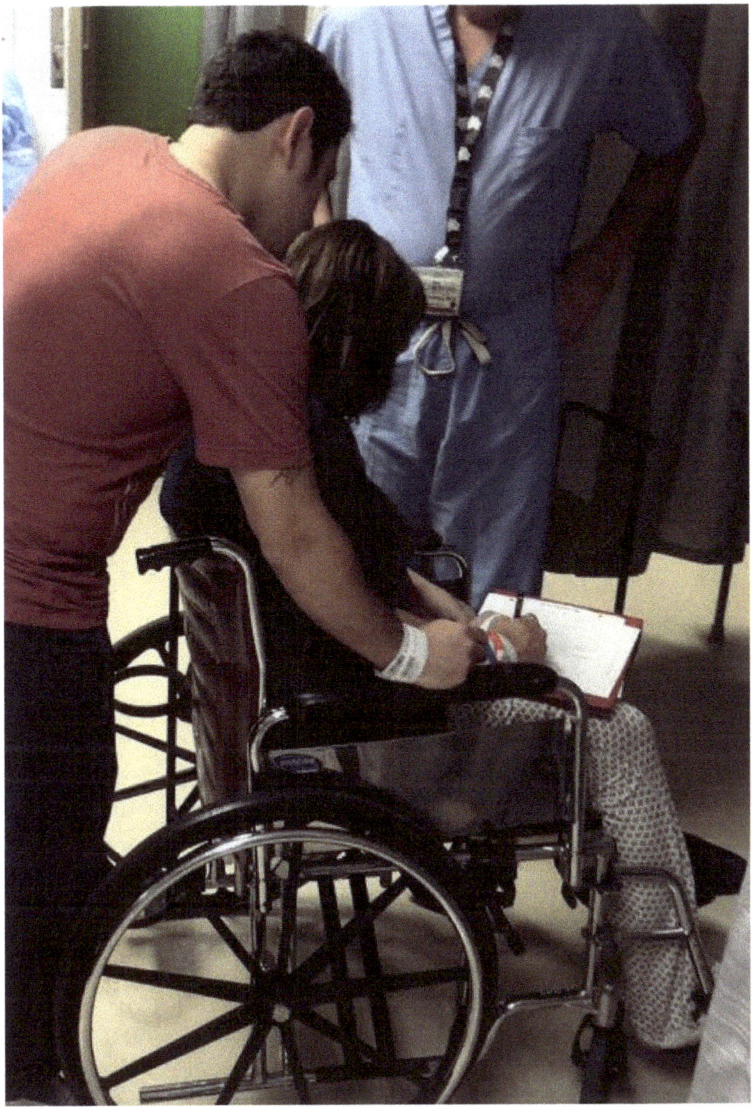

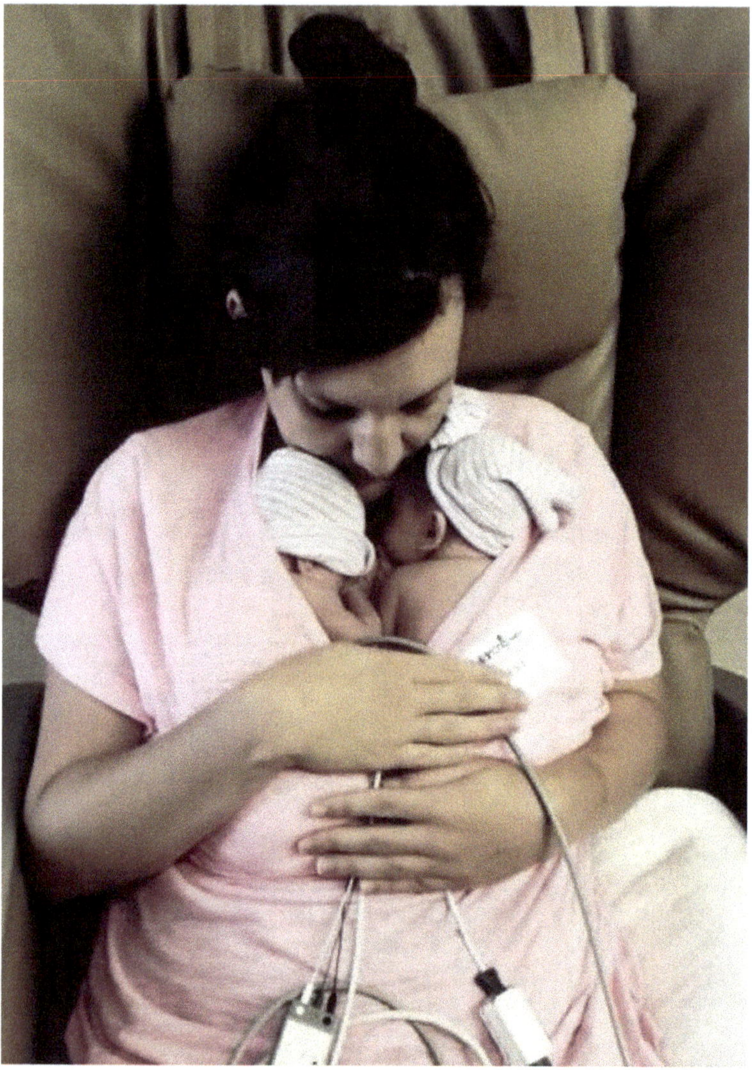

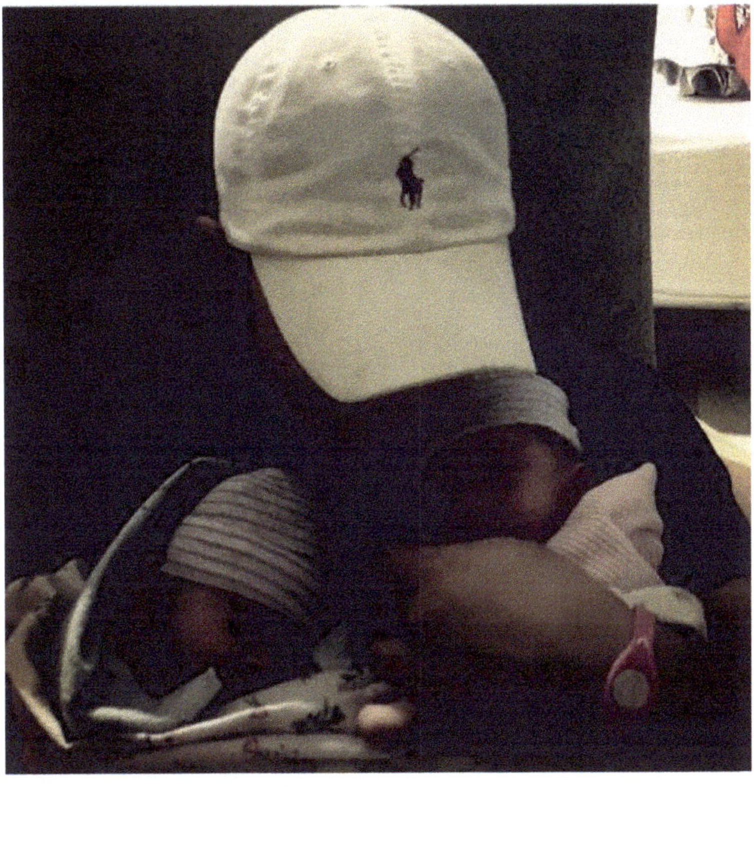

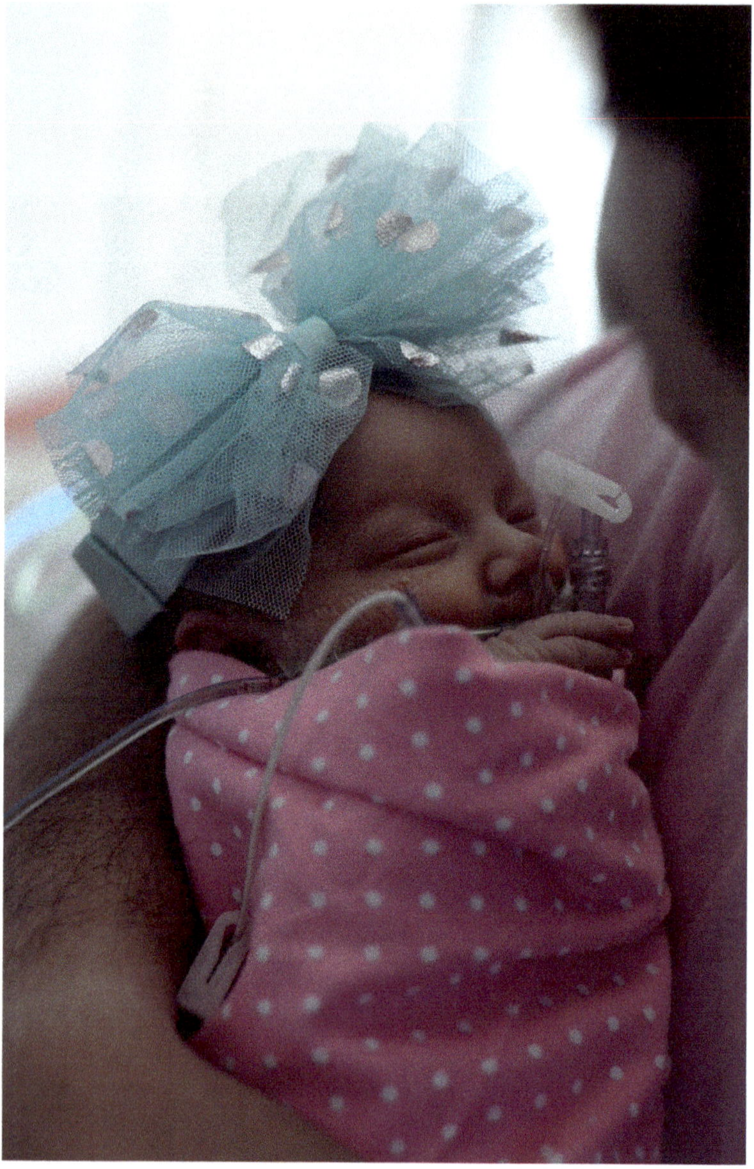

FIRST DAY HOME!

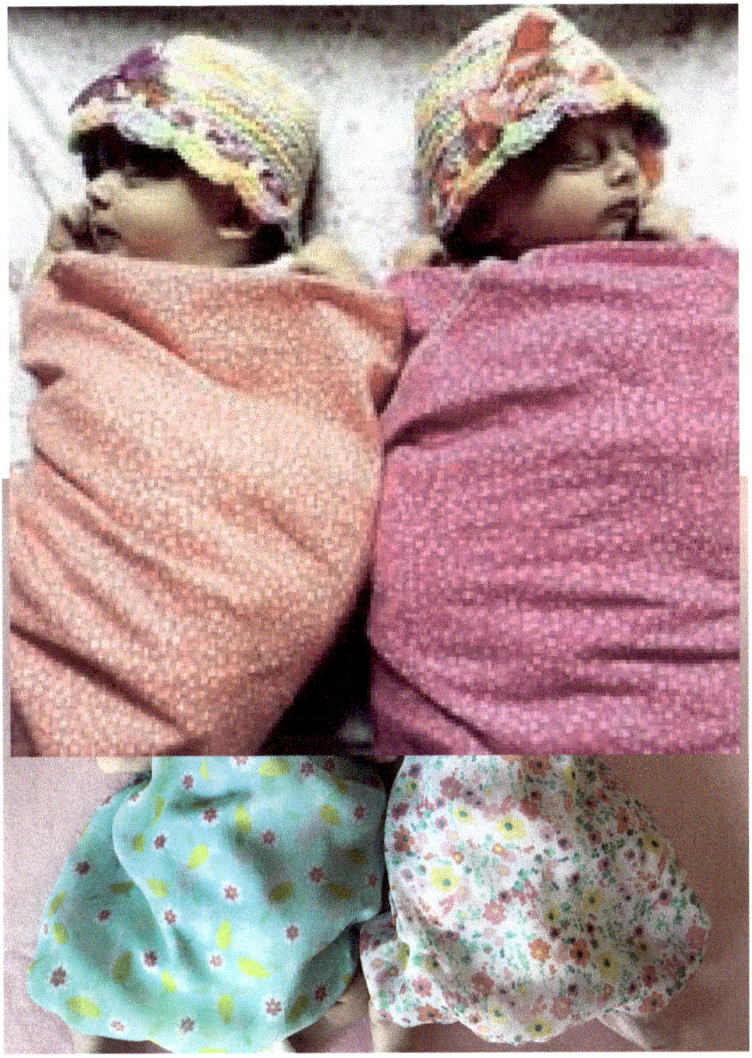

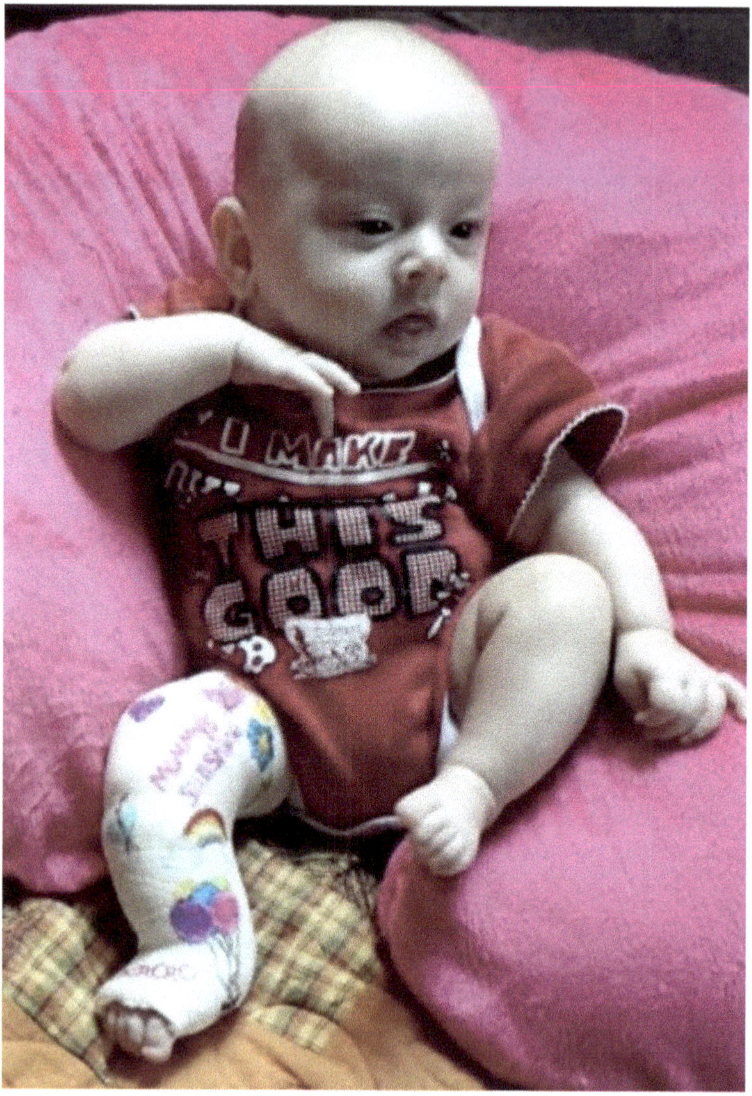

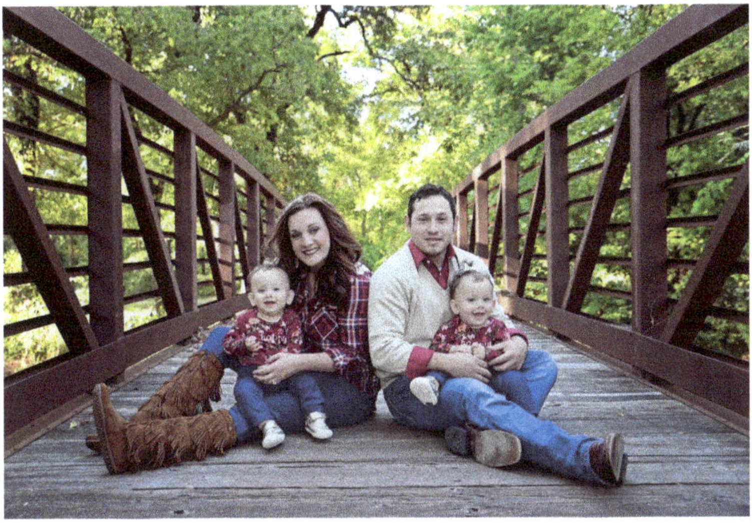

FIRST NIGHT APART

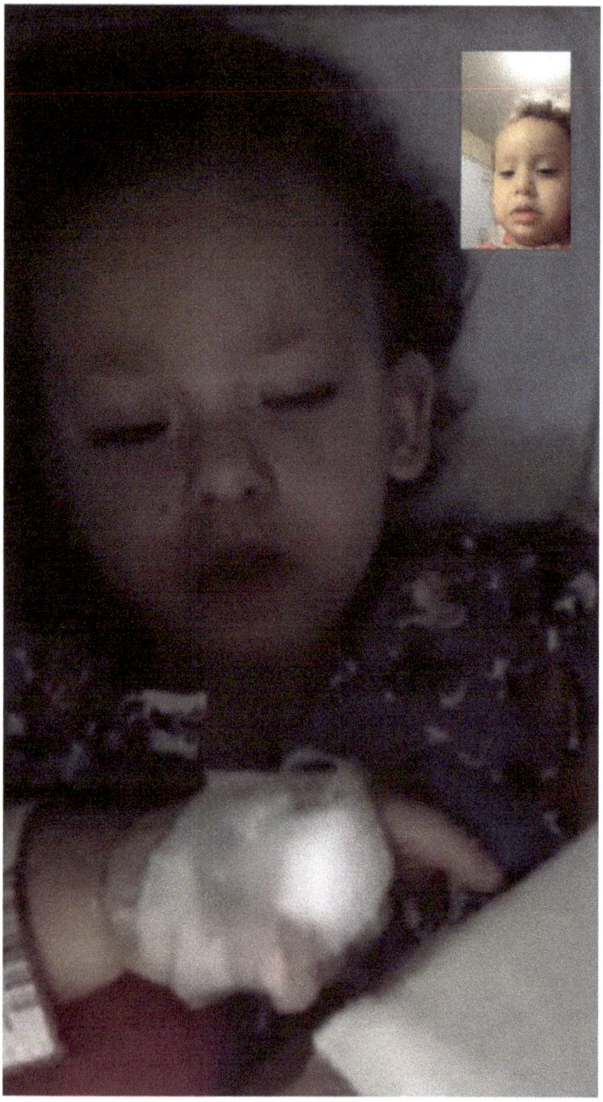

HARDWARE AFTER SURGERY. THEY HAD TO WEAR THIS FOR 5 WEEKS

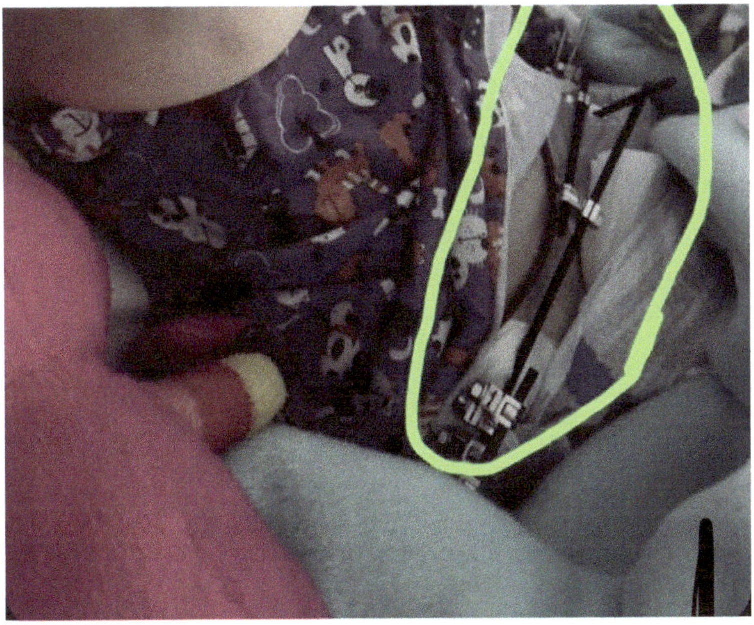

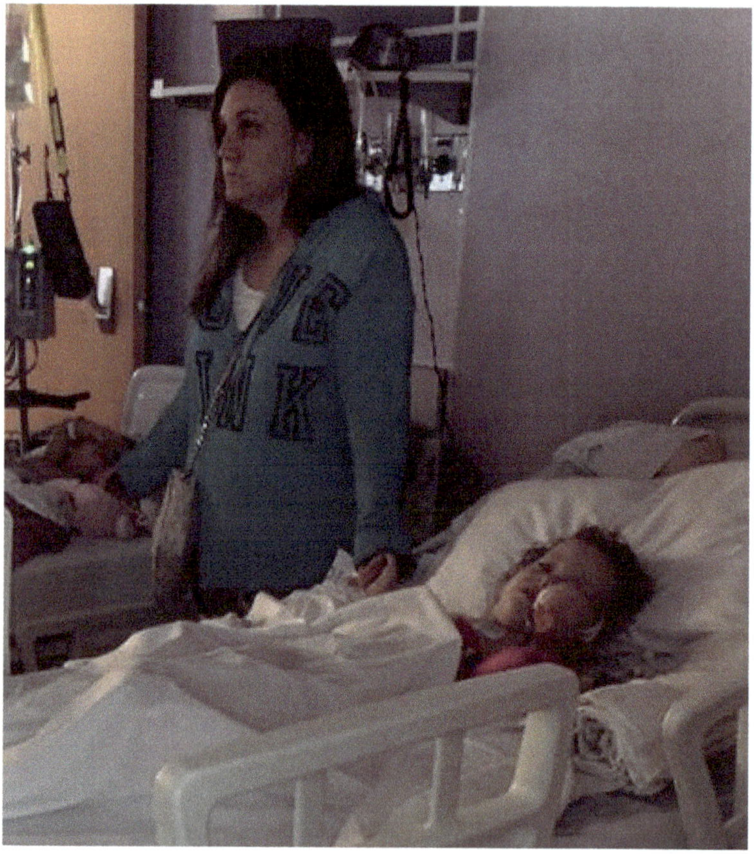

WALKING FROM THE APARTMENT TO THE HOSPITAL

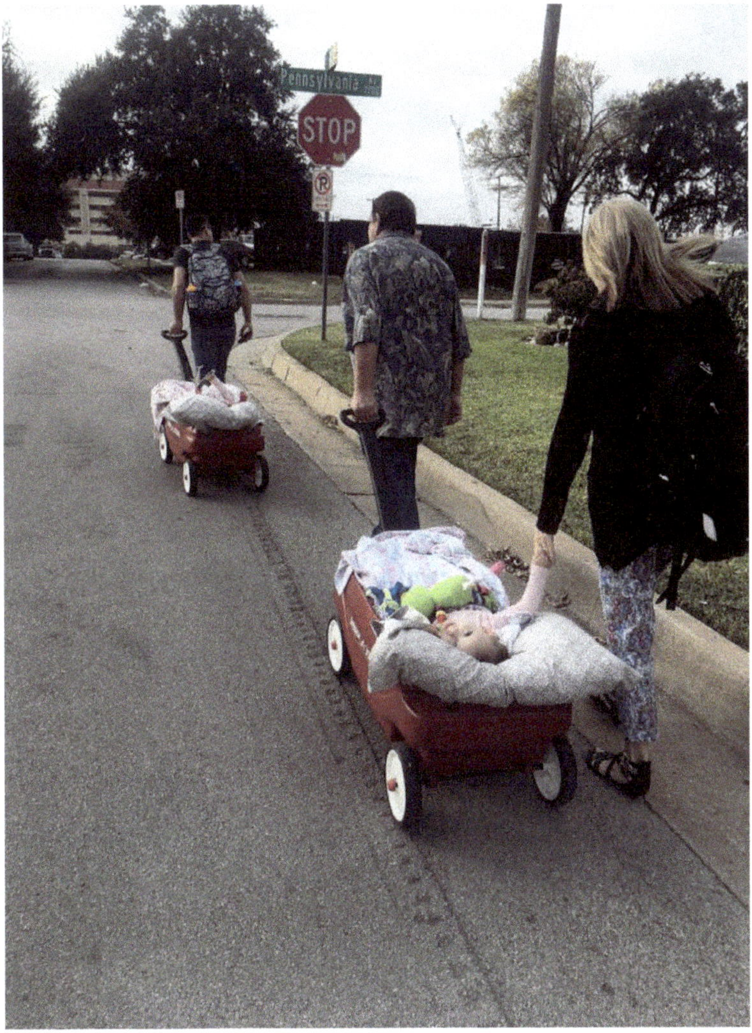

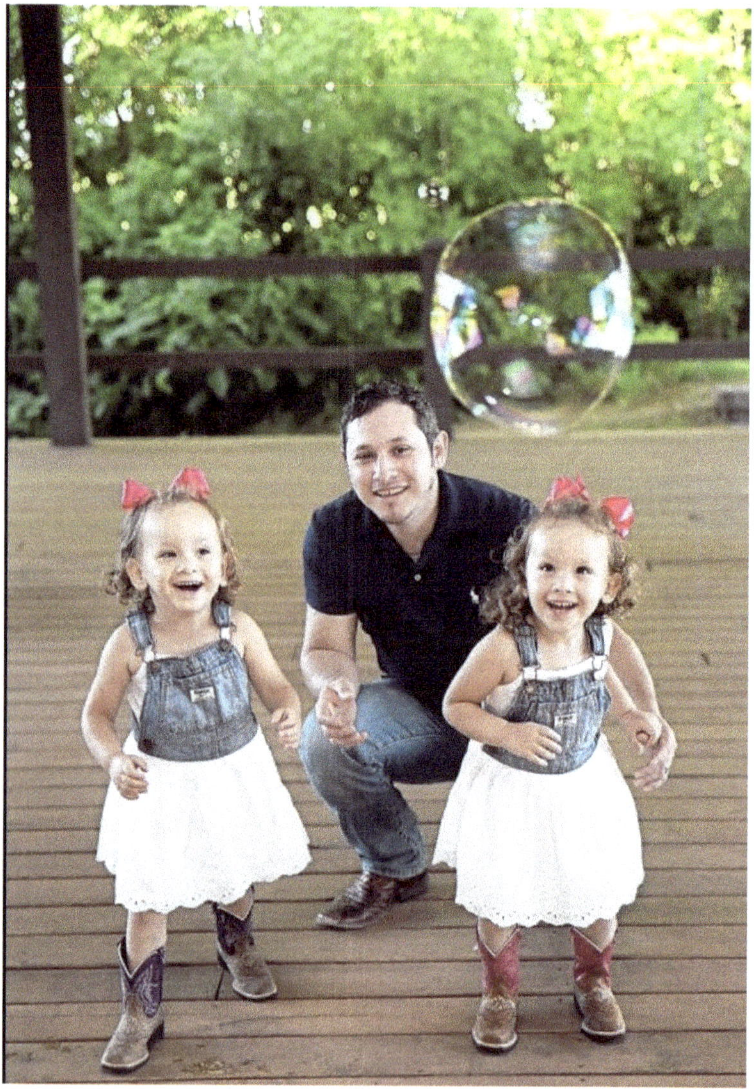

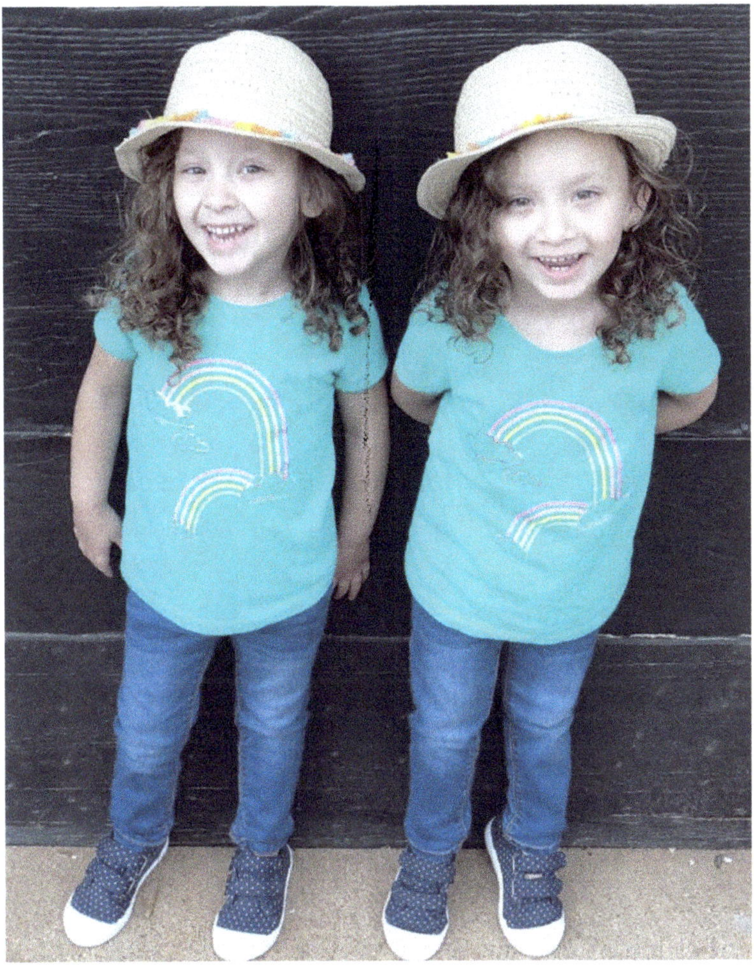

DADDY WALKING THE GIRLS TO THEIR FIRST DAY OF SCHOOL

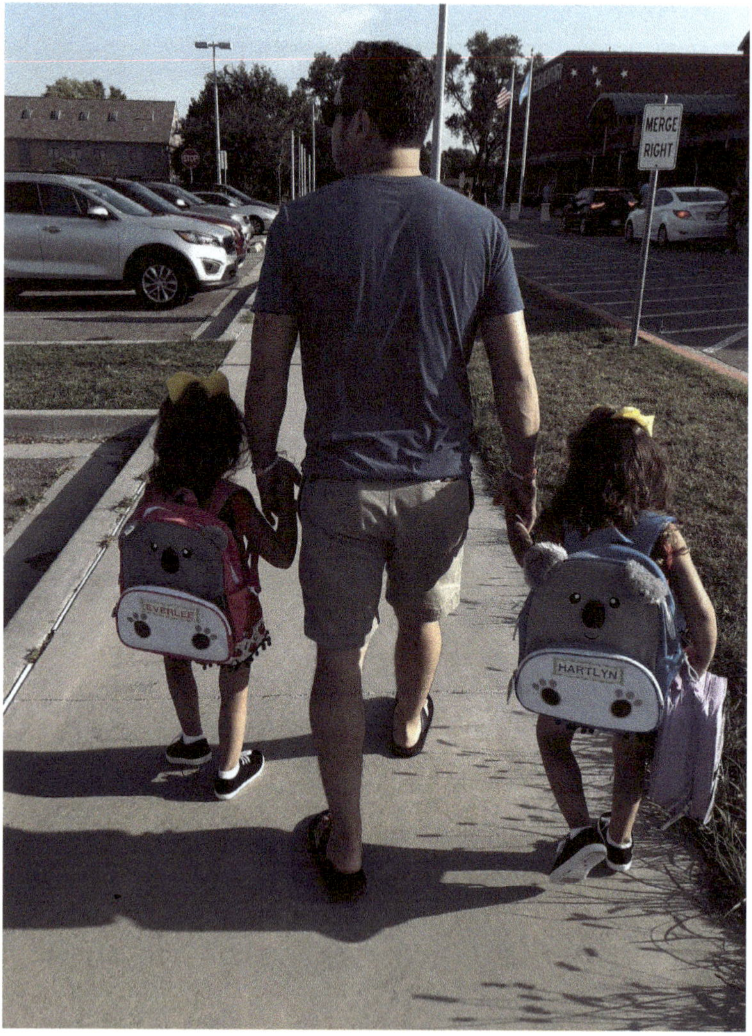

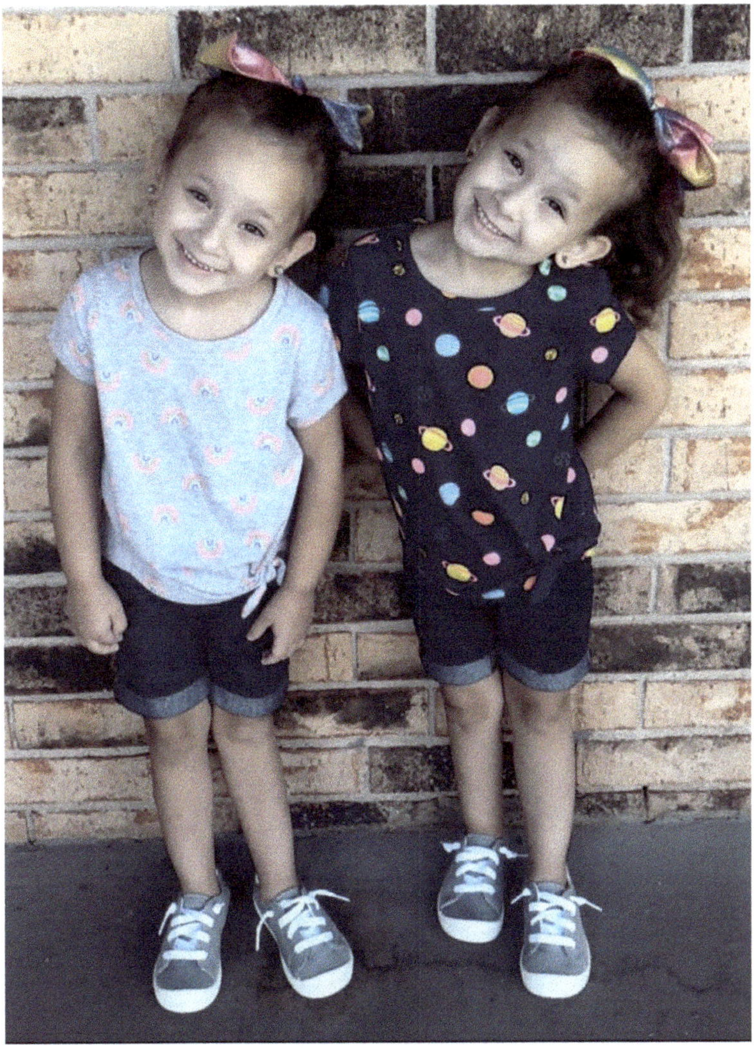

HARTLYN ON CAREER DAY

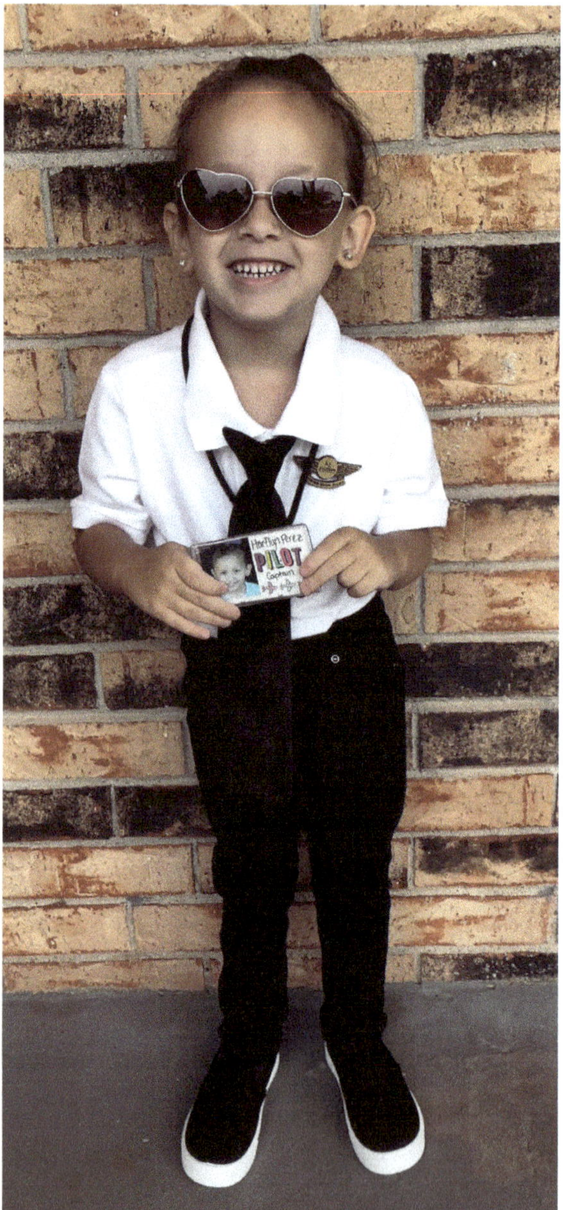

EVERLEE ON CAREER DAY

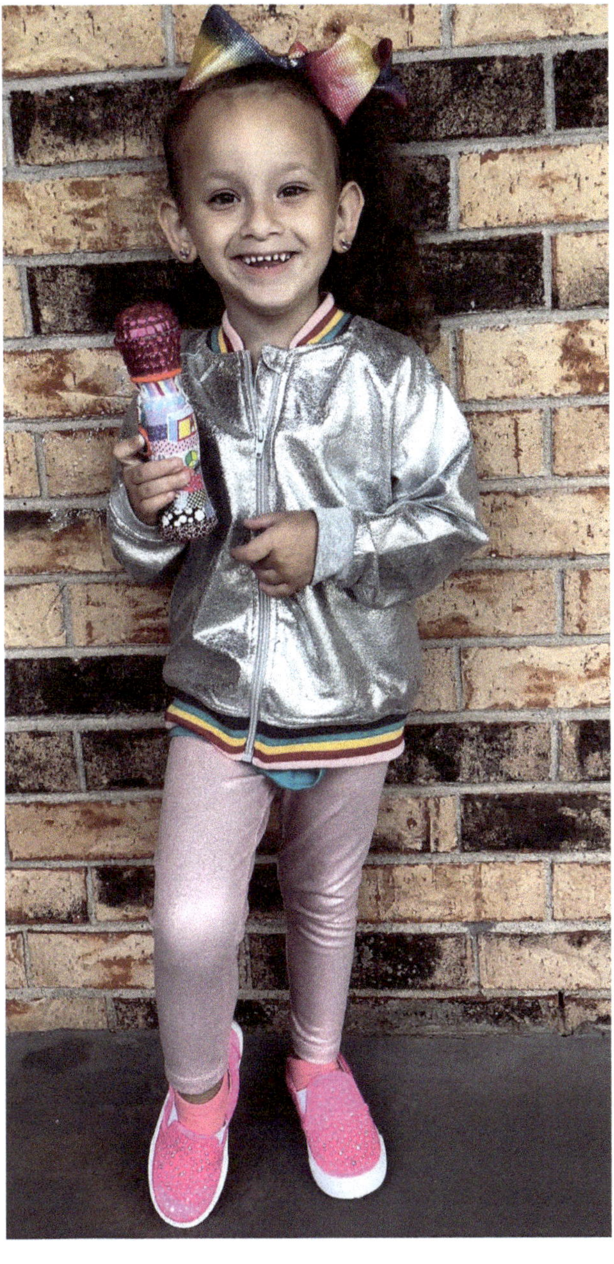

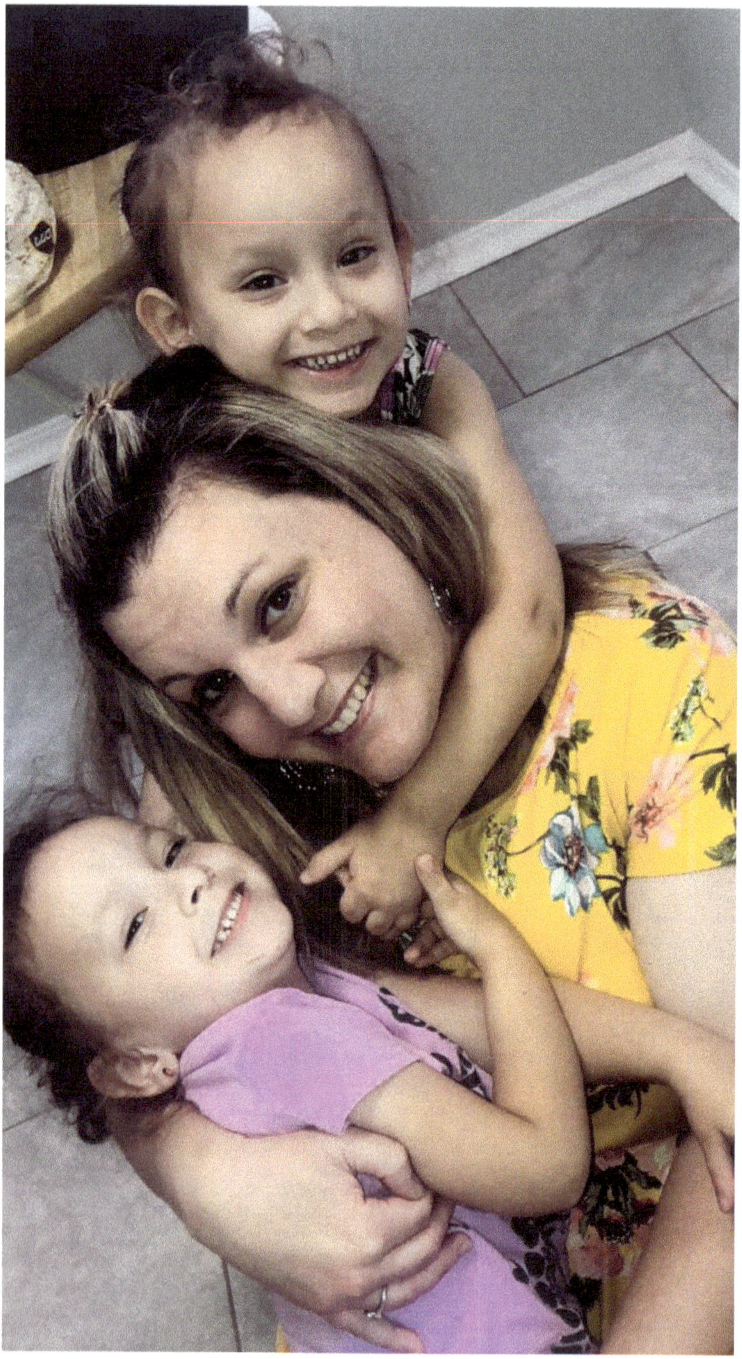

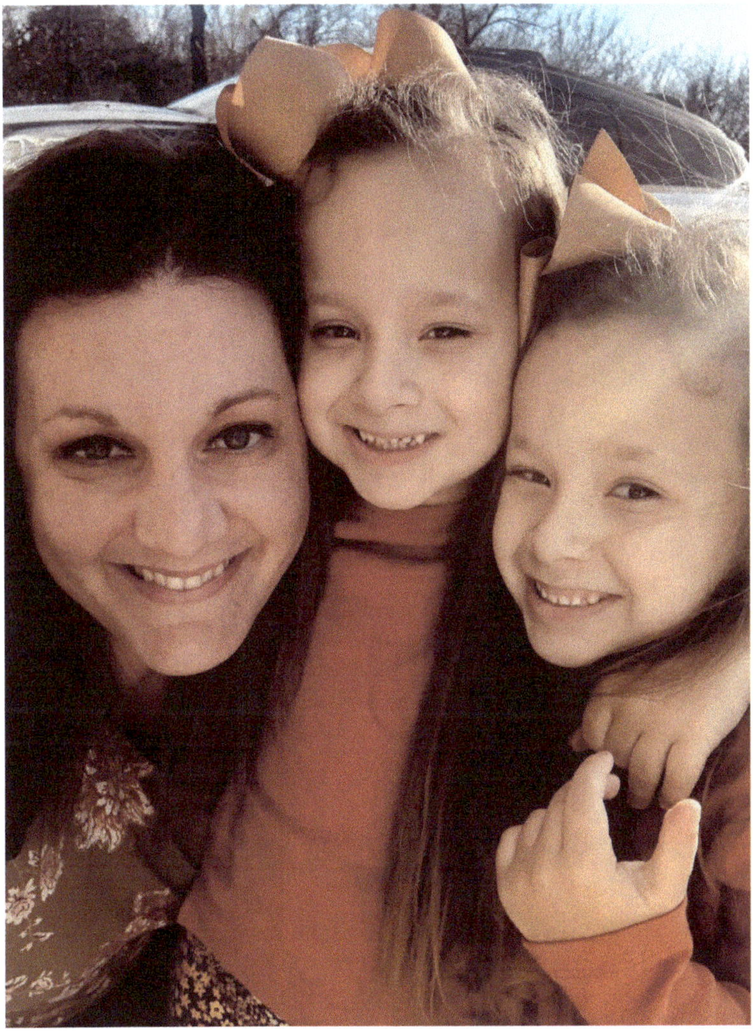

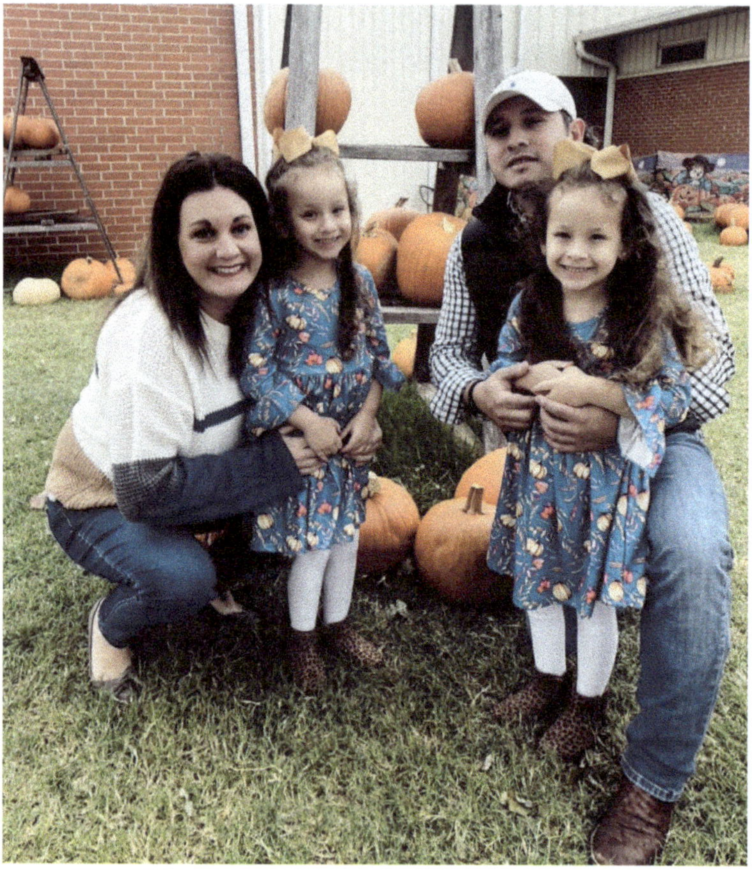

Milton Keynes UK
Ingram Content Group UK Ltd.
UKHW021817251023
431338UK00009B/70

9 781736 331811